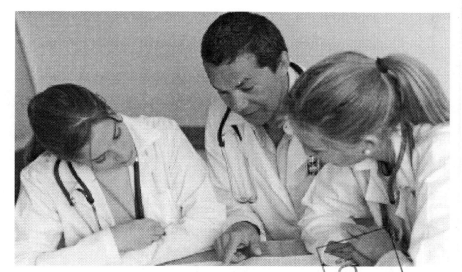

Effective Medical Teaching Skills

A practical guide to medical education

**Pervinder Bhogal, Gauraang Bhatnagar,
Maninder Bhogal, Tom Conner,
Shvaita Ralhan & Matt Green**

Edited by
Jane Young

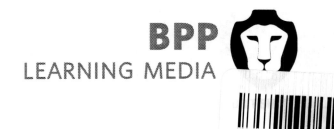

BPP
LEARNING MEDIA

First edition October 2011

ISBN 9781 4453 7955 5
e-ISBN 9781 4453 8584 6

British Library Cataloguing-in-Publication Data
A catalogue record for this book is available from
the British Library

Published by
BPP Learning Media Ltd
BPP House, Aldine Place
London W12 8AA

www.bpp.com/health

Typeset by Replika Press Pvt Ltd, India
Printed in the United Kingdom

Your learning materials, published by BPP
Learning Media Ltd, are printed on paper
sourced from sustainable, managed forests.

The views expressed in this book are those of BPP
Learning Media and not those of the NHS, NICE
or any other institute referenced in this book.
BPP Learning Media are in no way associated
with or endorsed by the NHS, NICE or any other
institute referenced in this book.

The contents of this book are intended as a guide
and not professional advice. Although every effort
has been made to ensure that the contents of
this book are correct at the time of going to
press, BPP Learning Media, the Editor and the
Author make no warranty that the information
in this book is accurate or complete and accept
no liability for any loss or damage suffered by
any person acting or refraining from acting as
a result of the material in this book.

Every effort has been made to contact the
copyright holders of any material reproduced
within this publication. If any have been
inadvertently overlooked, BPP Learning Media
will be pleased to make the appropriate credits
in any subsequent reprints or editions.

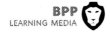

Contents

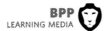

Contents

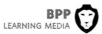

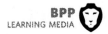

BPP
LEARNING MEDIA

About the Publisher

BPP Learning Media is dedicated to supporting aspiring professionals with top quality learning material. BPP Learning Media's commitment to success is shown by our record of quality, innovation and market leadership in paper-based and e-learning materials. BPP Learning Media's study materials are written by professionally-qualified specialists who know from personal experience the importance of top quality materials for success.

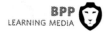

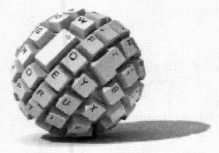

Free Companion Material

Readers can access practical exercises based on each chapter, which they can download to use in their teaching sessions, for free online.

To access the above companion material please visit **www.bpp.com/freehealthresources**

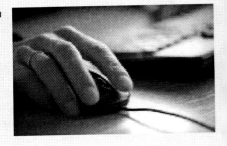

About the Authors

Dr Pervinder Bhogal is training to be an Interventional Neuroradiologist on the London Neuroradiology fellowship. He graduated from UCL Medical School in 2004 and completed his MRCS before entering Radiology. He has completed a Diploma in Medical Education and believes that all medical students can become great doctors with the right guidance and teaching.

Dr Gauraang Bhatnagar attended Guy's, King's and St Thomas' School of Medicine and graduated in 2004. After completing surgical training in London he joined the Southwest Peninsula Radiology Academy in 2008. He is a fellow of The Higher Education Academy, and has combined his interest in Radiology and Medical Education in a variety of publications over the last few years.

Dr Shvaita Ralhan trained at Guy's, King's and St Thomas' School of Medicine and graduated in 2004. After completing her core medical training in London she moved to the southwest of England and is a specialist trainee in General Internal Medicine and Geriatrics. Shvaita feels that understanding the basics of clinical education is an essential skill for all doctors. She is a fellow of The Higher Education Academy and is currently studying for a Masters degree in Clinical Education.

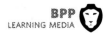

Contributors

Sagaar Mandavia
University Hospital of South Manchester

Dr Andy Brereton
Conquest Hospital, East Sussex

Dr Tom Booth and **Dr Yen Zhi Tang**
Royal Free Hospital, Hampstead

Dr Ynyr Hughes-Roberts
Addenbrooke's Hospital, Cambridge

Dr Sumanjit Gill
Royal London Hospital

Dr Prity Gupta
Bart's and The London NHS Trust

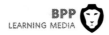

Acknowledgments (figures)

Figure 3.1 Representation of Knowles' andragogy showing the four postulates of adult learning
Adapted from APTECH Global Learning Solutions, reproduced under a Creative Commons Attribution Share-Alike License. http://leanlearning.wikispaces.com/instructional_design

Figure 4.1 The learning matrix
Adapted from Learning Styles: individualising computer based learning environments. Association for Learning Technology 3:53–62

Figure 5.1 Average retention rates for material taught using various methods
Adapted from National Training Laboratories Learning Pyramid.
www.bioscience.heacademy.ac.uk/journal/vol3/beej-3-5.aspx

Figure 5.3 A model of the spiral curriculum
Adapted from the Dundee Medical School model www.dundee.ac.uk/medschool/undergraduate/mbchb/spiral-curriculum/

Figure 5.4 The SPICES model
Adapted from Harden, Snowden and Dunn (1984)
www.resources.scalingtheheights.com/SPICES.htm

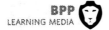

Dedications

To our friends and families for their support, love and enduring tolerance.

A special dedication to:

Emma Jayne Gumbleton

For all the smiles, laughter and beautiful memories, but most of all for being there when I needed you.

x x x

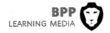

Foreword

The study and practice of good principles of medical education have come of age over the last few decades. No longer the province of an academic department, they have spilled over into all areas of medical teaching such that all teachers of both undergraduate medical students, and postgraduate doctors and paramedical staff are expected to have had some training in how to teach and assess. Many doctors actively pursue qualifications in medical education alongside their clinical and professional examinations. Students now expect to be taught by effective teachers, and can be vocal when teaching is not delivering what they need.

An enthusiastic teacher will aways be an asset to any teaching activity, particularly if equally knowledgeable and a good communicator, but for all teachers there are useful techniques that can be learnt. It is important to understand something about how adult students learn, how to help them learn and how to adapt teaching to specific situations. Similarly for assessment, 'how to make the punishment fit the crime' so to speak.

This small book aims to give concise information about all of the above, and includes a section on using new technology.

It will be useful to those who are new to medical education as a discipline, and will probably be 'dipped into' rather than read from cover to cover. However, for those considering doing a formal qualification in medical education it is a good overview of the subject.

Jane Young
MBBS MSc FRCR
Consultant Radiologist, Whittington Hospital, London
Honorary Senior Lecturer UCL / Royal Free Medical School
Regional Educational Advisor for the Royal College of
Radiologists
Previously: Director of Postgraduate Medical Education,
Whittington Hospital
Associate Dean for London Deanery

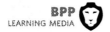

Preface

The word **'Doctor'** (n.) = one who teaches, or one who has been taught, comes from the Latin verb *to teach* (doceo, docere, docui, doctus).

As doctors we have a duty to teach and the UK General Medical Council has highlighted this essential role:

> *Every doctor who comes into contact with medical students should recognise the importance of role models in developing appropriate behaviours towards patients, colleagues and others. Doctors with particular responsibility for teaching students must develop the skills and practices of a competent teacher and must make sure that students are properly supervised.*

For previous generations of medical teachers there was little or no instruction in how to teach. If they were fortunate they had the example of good teachers, who they could follow, and memories of poor teachers, whose methods they tried to avoid. Excellence in teaching was a poor relation to research excellence. This is no longer the case, and it is customary for doctors in training to be asked for their experience of teaching, and to demonstrate formal training in teaching methods, including in job applications.

Being a good teacher is a rewarding experience in itself as is being a good clinician. Knowledge, skills and appropriate attitudes are required for both.

This book aims to provide the basic fundamentals of teaching theory alongside practical tips and advice for teachers at all stages of their careers. We have included exercises throughout the book in order to help gain the most from it.

We hope you find it helpful and of practical benefit. Most of all we hope that this book helps you on a lifelong journey to becoming an excellent teacher that your students remember fondly.

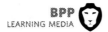

Chapter 1
Teaching is not learning

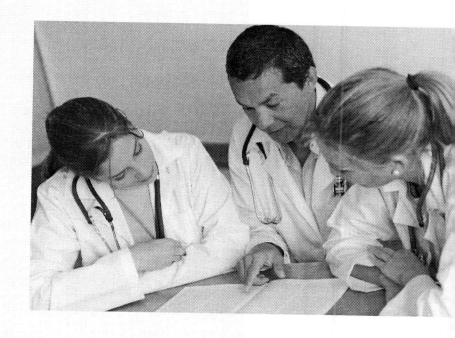

Teaching is not learning

Introduction

In order to understand how learning takes place it is helpful to be familiar with some of the theories of learning. In this chapter we discuss some of the more common and accepted theories of learning.

Theories of learning

Education can be defined as an experience that has a formative experience on an individual. The role of the teacher is to help facilitate this, and in medicine this most often refers to the act of imparting knowledge. To do this effectively a basic knowledge of the ways in which students learn is essential.

There are numerous theories about how learning occurs. An early philosophical branch of psychology popular in the early 19th century was behaviouralism. This was based on the theory that all actions, thoughts and feelings were 'behaviours' and hence were the reaction to a stimulus. This school of thought was influenced by the famous classical conditioning experiments of Ivan Pavlov. While elements of this apply to teaching methods (such as praising a correct response to a question reinforcing learning) its popularity was overtaken by 'cognitive theory' in the 20th century.

The 'cognitive' movement of the 1950s brought a new approach to psychology. It rejected introspection outcomes (as used by Freud) in favour of an acceptance of internal mental states (previously rejected by behaviourists). The term 'cognitive therapy' was coined by Ulric Neisser (1967) whose work proposed humans as 'information processing machines'. He stated that ' "cognition" refers to all processes by which the sensory input is transformed, reduced, elaborated, stored, recovered, and used'.

These theories have been built on by constructivist cognitive theories. The basis of this movement, often attributed to the work of Jean Piaget, is that there is an existing framework of knowledge and this can be added to by two processes, assimilation and accommodation. Assimilation is the process by which further information is added

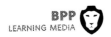

to the existing framework, without changing it. Accommodation occurs when the basic mental framework needs to change – for example when something fails unexpectedly.

Piaget also coined the term 'schema' – a mental structure that with respect to education can be loosely thought of as representing building blocks. Elements of this theory are evident in modern teaching methods – for example by presenting information that the students should already know before or early in a lecture is a way of activating the relevant knowledge enabling further schema to be added or altered more easily.

 Pause for thought
Consider lectures you have attended. Do you recognise elements of these theories of learning in the teaching methods used?

Types of learning

Many skill sets are used in the practice of clinical medicine. A major focus of current medical teaching is to encourage the development of problem-solving skills to be used in diagnostic situations. There are various ways of tackling diagnostic problems and a combination is often used to reach the best answer. These techniques include: pattern recognition, understanding of basic scientific and medical concepts and knowledge of causes of symptoms and signs (eg lists of categories of disease or causes of pathology).

Pioneering research into types of learning at higher education institutions by Marton, Entwistle and Ramsden and others in the late 1970s and early 1980s focused on students' perspectives of teaching. They developed the theory that there were two fundamentally different types of learning that students adopted – 'surface' learning and 'deep' learning. Surface learning describes the learning of facts and material, sometimes apparently unrelated ,whilst 'deep' learning describes a more analytical approach to learning where there is an understanding of concepts, rather than facts in isolation, relating the new knowledge to previous knowledge, everyday experience, and organising it into a coherent structure.

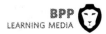

Pause for thought
- How often have you faced an exam where you learnt lists of facts but on passing still felt you did not understand the material?
- Which material did you really feel you completely understood as a student? Was this taught or examined differently?

Although being a doctor requires a knowledge of a large number of facts (in comparison to other subjects such as art subjects or science courses where conceptual theories appear to be more central to the curriculum) it is essential that the clinician has an abilty to analyse complex information. Thus deep learning is important to develop a critical and scientific approach to thinking and improve the analytical skills required for solving complex clinical problems.

Whether surface or deep learning occurs will partly depend on both how the subject is taught and how the assessment of the knowledge is made. Lectures consisting of slides of long lists of facts with an end of term examination involving regurgitation of these facts will only convince the student that simple memorisation of these lists is the desirable achievement. To engage and encourage students to use high order in learning is a challenge in any subject. This is exacerbated by the breadth of knowledge which medicine encompasses and the necessary time constraints for covering each subject.

 Practical points
- Review a recent teaching session or lecture you gave.
- What proportion of the lesson was dedicated to superficial learning and what proportion was dedicated to trying to encourage a deep learning of the subject?
- Do you think you managed to achieve enough deep learning processes?
- How could this be improved next time?

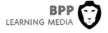

Metacognition

However able a teacher may be in conveying knowledge and ideas to students, the goal may be hampered by the ability of their students to learn. This is influenced by the way in which they learn as much as their academic ability.

The ability to think about one's own cognitive processes – 'thinking about thinking' – is known as metacognition. The term metacognition was first used by J H Flavell (1979). He describes it as:

> *Metacognition refers to one's knowledge concerning one's own cognitive processes or anything related to them, eg, the learning-relevant properties of information or data. For example, I am engaging in metacognition if I notice that I am having more trouble learning A than B; if it strikes me that I should double check C before accepting it as fact.*

Flavell broadly divided metacognition into four components:

- Metacognitive knowledge/awareness – what someone understands about their own or others' cognitive processes
- Metacognitive experiences – these provide a resource of previous learning experiences
- Goals and tasks – the desired outcome
- Strategies – the ability to regulate cognitive functions through various activities and to be able to match the correct strategies for different tasks

Helping students develop this ability enables them to be better students, particularly in complex situations, which applies to much of the medical knowledge they are expected to gain. Many may already have developed effective strategies, but they can still benefit from this. Even highly intelligent students may benefit as they encounter academically harder problems than they have been used to previously.

Being an effective learner involves making a plan to learn, setting goals, monitoring how the learning is progressing and adapting or changing strategies if necessary. This is a continuous cycle, much like a 'feedback loop'.

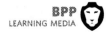

Our individual beliefs about our ability to learn influences how successful we are at learning. There is evidence to show that those students who believe they can learn, often with perseverance (as opposed to those who believe the particular subject or task is too difficult, for example) do better.

So helping students set goals, giving them opportunities to 'monitor' or 'test' their understanding and their knowledge, and offering different strategies for learning, can help them. For example – using mnemonics where appropriate, encouraging practice of certain types of problems.

 Practical points

The use of metacognitive skills can be encouraged by your methods of teaching, for example:

- Verbalising what the teacher is thinking when explaining ideas or solving problems.
- Explaining a desired thought process or model when encountering a problem (for example when thinking of a list of differential diagnoses and balancing those more probable versus less).
- Giving examples of your own metacognitive methods (for example use of rhymes or mnemonics).
- Setting tasks that encourage self regulation.

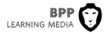

Key points

- Models of learning include behaviouralist, cognitive, and constructive theories that have influenced modern teaching methods.
- If a deep analytical approach to learning is required the teaching and assessment must be designed to encourage this.
- Students do not always have the necessary metacognitive skills required for a critical approach to learning and should be encouraged to develop these.

References

Entwistle, N J & Ramsden, P (1983) *Understanding Student Learning* (Croom Helm)

Flavell, J H (1979). Metacognition and Cognitive Monitoring: A new Area of Cognitive-Developmental Inquiry, *American Psychologist*, 34, 906–911

Marton, F & Saljo, R (1976) On Qualitative Differences in Learning, *British Journal of Educational Psychology*, 46, pp. 4–11 & 115–127

Neisser, U (1967) *Cognitive Psychology* (New York: Appleton-Century-Crofts)

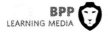

Chapter 2

What is learning? Knowledge, skills, and attitudes

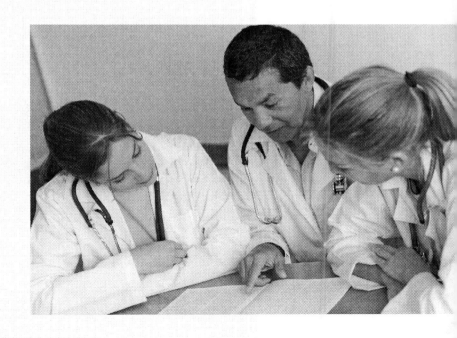

What is learning? Knowledge, skills, and attitudes

Introduction

Learning is not simply the rote regurgitation of facts learned from a dusty textbook. Learning in medicine occurs continuously at a conscious and subconscious level. In this chapter we look more closely at learning.

Formal and informal learning

While the formal educational curriculum is normally delivered by lectures and structured tutorials, there are a myriad of learning experiences that occur elsewhere. Within medicine for example, experience may be gained from: listening to interactions between working doctors, ad hoc teaching sessions on hospital wards, or from talking to patients and family members. These *informal* learning experiences are of vital importance and can form a significant amount of the overall learning at an educational institution such as a medical school.

 Pause for thought

- What types of informal learning did you experience in medical school?
- How did the knowledge gained from informal education experiences differ from that gained from formal learning? How important was it?
- How much of your current medical knowledge can you attribute to informal learning?

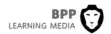

The 'hidden curriculum' – includes skills, attitudes and behaviour

What is the role of education? The obvious answer includes the acquisition of knowledge – yet knowledge is only one of the many desirable qualities of a doctor. For a doctor a wide range of other skills, including social skills, are vital, for example, good interpersonal communication skills with colleagues and patients and an appropriate attitude towards work (punctuality, working hard etc). How do we learn this and can it be taught?

Informal learning of social skills occurs from an early age for example, from praise or discipline received from parents or peers when copying or rejecting socially acceptable behavioural patterns. Primary and secondary school education systems indirectly further this learning in what has been described as the 'hidden curriculum'. This term is credited to Phillip Jackson from his book *Life in Classrooms* (1968). Through observations of public classrooms in the USA he noted that schools do more than simply impart knowledge. They actively encourage and reward social and behavioural skills such as waiting quietly, co-operating, being punctual, showing deference to seniority (eg peers and teachers). At the same time it was argued by Robert Dreeben (1968) that family life alone did not sufficiently prepare children for the adult world. He concluded that schooling causes children to 'form transient social relationships, submerge much of their personal identity, and accept the legitimacy of categorical treatment' – all skills necessary for the adult workplace.

Hafferty (1998) summarised these ideas within the context of medical education by describing 'the notion of a multidimensional learning environment with at least three interrelated spheres of influence'. These were:

* The stated and formally endorsed curriculum
* The interpersonal ad hoc teaching between teachers – the informal curriculum
* The organisational infrastructure that influences learning and socialisation to the normal professional culture – the hidden curriculum

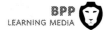

An appreciation of the ability to learn from formal, informal and hidden curricula helps us understand that we all have the capacity to learn from every experience. To fully realise this potential requires self-critical appraisal and awareness of all learning experiences both as a teacher and a student. This skill can serve you throughout your medical career. An example of this would be critically assessing how well you dealt with an upset patient, comparing your outcomes with those of your colleagues and adapting your strategies accordingly.

 Practical points

- Make a list of the objectives you want your students to learn prior to the teaching session — both from the hidden and the normal curriculum.
- Think of the skills, attitudes and behaviours your students could learn from watching you interact with patients. For example how do you introduce yourself, structure your questions, how is the patient seated, how do you adjust eye contact throughout a consultation? When watching a student take a history — do they do these unspoken things appropriately?

 Key points

- Not all learning takes place in a formal learning environment.
- We also learn social skills and attributes through a hidden curriculum.
- Every experience can be a learning opportunity.

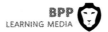

References

Dreeben, R (1968) 'What is learned in classrooms?' *On What is Learned in School.* (London: Addison-Wesley)

Hafferty FW (1998) 'Beyond Curriculum Reform: Confronting Medicine's Hidden Curriculum', *Acad Med*; 73:403–407

Jackson, P (1968) *Life in Classrooms* (New York: Holt, Reinhart & Winston)

Margolis, E (ed.) (2001) *The Hidden Curriculum in Higher Education* (New York & London: Routledge)

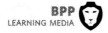

Chapter 3

Understanding the needs of the learner

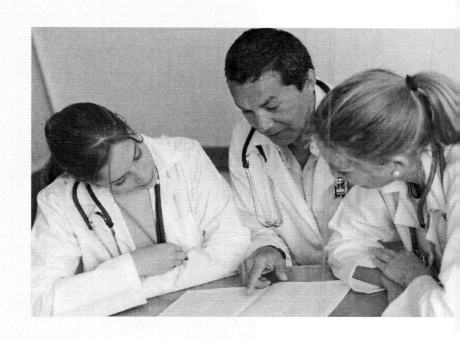

Understanding the needs of the learner

Introduction

What is the difference between 'training' and 'education'? Is there a difference?

Training is a form of learning undertaken to achieve a specific goal or acquire a specific skill. It is usually measured against a set standard; when you've reached the standard, you are considered trained.

In its Latin origin, education means 'leading out.' Strictly speaking, education is about developing a person's potential, helping them to discover the abilities that they have and giving them the tools to use them. However it is usually used to mean the whole system of imparting knowledge, ethics and culture; it includes **both** learning and training.

The adult learner – what's different?

 Pause for thought

How different are you as a learner now compared to, say, when you were working for school exams? Perhaps note down some of these differences.

Recognising that every learner is an individual, with their own set of needs and experiences, is essential to becoming a good teacher. Increased awareness of a learner's needs is essential to moving away from the traditional didactic form of teaching and the development of a partnership between teacher and student.

The adult learner differs in a number of fundamental ways to a child who is learning (see below).

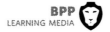

Children as learners	Adults as learners
Subject centered	Problem centered
Predominantly driven by external motivators	Predominantly driven by internal motivators
Less confident at challenging and analysing taught material; more open, malleable and adaptable	More confident when challenging and analysing taught material; may reject ideas that contradict their own beliefs
Have less life experience to discuss and draw ideas from	Willing to discuss previous experience and mistakes
Have fewer other responsibilities	Have many other responsibilities in their lives
Have fewer pre-formed habits/ views	Have traditional views
Play a more submissive role	Play a more active role
Less goal and relevance orientated	More goal and relevance orientated

Table 3.1 Important differences between adult and child learners

It is important as doctors teaching adults that we are aware of these differences and adapt our teaching accordingly. Adult learners usually have prior experience that they refer to. This may be transferrable or relevant to their current learning. In fact experience is central to how an adult learns. It is often through reflection on an experience, that new skills and knowledge are acquired by adults, particularly doctors. Therefore, encouraging reflection is an essential part of the process of teaching adults. Adult learners can be an active contributor to the learning process and often this enriches the experience for the educator! However, they may require an explanation of why they need to learn certain material, and how (on a more practical level) it will help them in a specific scenario. Adult learners are more self-directed in their learning style and as a teacher it is essential to encourage and match this. Your style of teaching may need to be more as a 'facilitator' (helping them learn) rather than an authority delivering your expertise. Paternalism in an adult educational experience is rarely useful.

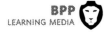

Motivations for learning

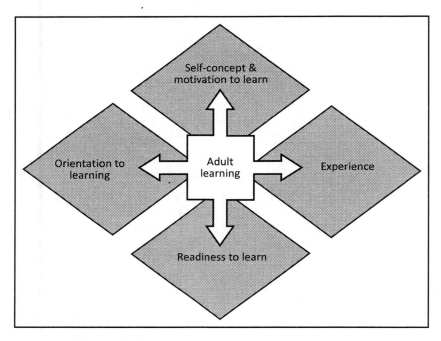

Figure 3.1 Representation of Knowles' andragogy showing the four postulates of adult learning (adapted from APTECH Global Learning Solutions, reproduced under a Creative Commons Attribution Share-Alike License: http://leanlearning.wikispaces.com instructional_design)

Motivation is regarded as a prerequisite for learning. If students are motivated then learning occurs at a more efficient rate. Motivating students can be one of the biggest challenges we face as teachers.

Extrinsic motivations are sometimes regarded as being less powerful, yet still play an important role:

* Providing a qualification that contributes to career progression
* Building their CV
* Gaining recognition

Intrinsic motivators are more powerful as drivers and these are outlined below (Manlone and Lepper 1987, Bullock *et al.* 2008).

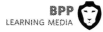

- Students may increase their self-esteem through their success.
- Students may curious to investigate other ways of doing things, and learn about things they do not know about.
- The material they learn will be useful in their daily working lives.
- The material is interesting and intriguing.
- They wish to challenge themselves.
- They wish to gain independence in skills to move towards autonomy.
- The process of learning is fun.
- They have desires for social comparison (comparing their performance against that of others).

Most people in a medical setting possess a combination of intrinsic and extrinsic motivators to their learning.

Developing motivation in students that are unmotivated is very challenging and unfortunately there is no quick-fix. Encouraging and maintaining motivation in a student is important. To achieve this requires taking the following key factors into consideration.

Feedback

One of the ways of avoiding poor motivation is by supplying high quality feedback. Failure to achieve what is expected tends to demotivate a student. However, if an explanation of why failure occurred is given and how to improve performance in the future, the student is less likely to get demotivated by the experience (Fry, Ketteridge and Marshall 1999).

Assessment systems

Most students start courses and years of study highly motivated and tend to develop deep approaches to learning. However, as exams and assessments approach they become motivated by this extrinsic factor and develop surface approaches to learning (Entwistle 1998). If this method leads to success this is unlikely to change. It has therefore been suggested that assessment methods that encourage the use of deep learning are the most beneficial – such as case studies and problem solving, where acquired knowledge needs to be applied.

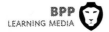

Combining these with some form of continuous assessment will hopefully encourage intrinsic factors of motivation.

'Self-regulatory' strategies

Students utilise their own methods to increase their motivation when they feel it is low. These include reminding themselves of the reward (eg qualification), changing the environment where learning/studying is taking place (eg taking regular breaks and working in a group) and cognitional strategies such as making and reading their own notes.

Personal development plans

Personal development plans (PDPs) are a great way to identify one's own learning needs and serve to focus our motivation and provide structure to our learning. There are many definitions for personal development plans, but in general it is a structured and supported process to assist students in arranging their own educational and career progression. It gives students the opportunity to reflect upon their own learning, performance, experiences and achievements (Jackson 2001, Fry, Ketteridge and Marshall 999). Nowadays PDPs form a mandatory part of the NHS eportfolio system which all doctors have to utilise once they qualify. Many universities also encourage students to make PDPs.

To some PDPs may seem like yet another paper exercise of little benefit to their learning. However, a well thought out PDPs can help to (Harvey 2009):

- Encourage development of self-directed learning.
- Improve planning and career management skills.
- Encourage lifelong learning.
- Promote understanding of how their learning relates to the wider context (especially useful in programmes that are modular).
- Help to construct goals that are valuable to an individual.
- Promote forward planning.
- When reviewed to an appropriate timescale, identify areas where there has (or has not) been progress.
- Can aid CV writing if used regularly.

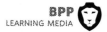

By understanding the benefits of PDPs you can, as a teacher, encourage students to use them as a tool to improve their learning and development.

Styles of learning and learning theories

As educators it is important that we have some understanding of how people learn, so that we can design and implement teaching that enhances the education of our students. There are two major schools of thought regarding learning. The first is that exemplified by Ivan Pavlov's and BF Skinner's models of classical and operant conditioning. This focuses on reinforcement to acquire skills. The second view is that of cognitive learning processes which involve not only acquisition of knowledge but also application of this knowledge, problem solving and decision making.

The Experiential Learning Model states that there are four parts to this cycle (Kolb 1984):

- Concrete experience (feeling)
- Reflective observation (watching)
- Abstract conceptualisation (thinking)
- Active experimentation (doing)

We all have individual ways of dealing with life and the problems it throws at us. Some rush in, others may carefully weigh things up, discuss with their friends. In the same way, we all have unique approaches to learning. Kolb went on to use this model to show that learners have different preferences within this cycle and developed four learning styles, each combining two parts of the cycle:

- Diverging (concrete experience and reflective observation)
- Assimilating (abstract conceptualisation and reflective observation)
- Converging (active conceptualisation and active experimentation)
- Accommodating (concrete experience and active experimentation)

David Kolb's model is useful as it not only offers us understanding about differing learning styles, but also an explanation of the cycle

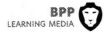

of learning which applies to us all. In fact Kolb designed a Learning Style inventory that can be used to deduce an individual's own learning style.

 Pause for thought

- What is your favoured learning style? Complete the Learning Style inventory and find out how you learn best (www.learning-styles-online.com)
- Compare with someone else's style. Is this a surprise?

There is arguably a strong similarity between the Honey and Mumford (1982) styles / stages and the corresponding Kolb learning styles:

Activist = Accommodating
Reflector = Diverging
Theorist = Assimilating
Pragmatist = Converging

Further description including the type of learner, how they learn most effectively and least effectively are summarised in Table 3.2.

Type of learner	Description	Most effective learning methods	Least effective learning methods
Theorist	• Collects and organises information • Enjoys exploring connections between ideas and concepts • Comfortable with objective facts	• Problem solving • Discussion • Reading and evaluating books	• Exploratory project work • Skills training

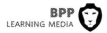

Type of learner	Description	Most effective learning methods	Least effective learning methods
Reflector	• Enjoys collecting data • Considers all perspectives • Takes a back seat in discussions • Learns from listening • Enjoys working alone	• Project work • Lectures • Independent study	• Spontaneous activity
Pragmatist	• Down to earth • Practical • Enjoys relating theory to practice • Enjoys clear guidelines	• Work-based projects • Practical problem solving	• Theoretical discussion
Activist	• Open-minded • Enjoys new challenges and experience • Likes being the centre of attention	• Group work • Discussions • Work shops	• Lectures • Reading alone

Table 3.2 Types of learners and preferred methods of teaching to assist their learning

The VARK classification of learning styles is one of the most popular classifications as it is the simplest. It represents our learning styles using sensory modalities and divides learners into visual, auditory and kinesthetic categories. Learners tend to utalise all modalities to acquire new information and experiences. However, according to the VARK modality theory, one or two of these receiving styles is dominant. However, it is important to note this style may not always be the same for **all** tasks. The learner may prefer one style of learning for one task, and a combination of others for a different task.

Knowing a person's (and your own) learning style enables learning to be orientated according to the preferred method. That said, everyone responds to and needs the stimulus of all types of learning styles to one extent or another – it's a matter of using an emphasis that fits best with the given situation and a individual's learning style preferences.

Encouraging a safe environment

The environment we create for learning is pivotal to our student's experience and how effective the learning process is. There are many facets that make up the environment we create, from the venue to the support you show your students.

The optimal learning environment:

- Encourages students to be active participants in their own education.
- Promotes and facilitates the student's discovery of the personal meaning of ideas.
- Encourages autonomy in the student.
- Provides a protected place where mistakes can be made and reflected upon.
- Establishes respect for the student.
- Encourages self-evaluation from the student.

It has been shown that there is a hierarchy of needs to be considered when learning (Maslow 1970). At the base of this are the basic physiological needs and as you move up the needs become more complex. For effective learning the most basic needs must be fulfilled in order to progress and achieve the next level. When teaching, it is important to consider this hierarchy.

Physiological needs

These needs are the most basic and include shelter, food, warmth and water. When planning a teaching episode ensure the venue is selected appropriately for the number of students. Plan regular breaks for students to use the toilets and have refreshments. Set the temperature and lighting so the room is comfortable to work in.

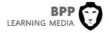

Safety need

This encompasses the student's need to be safe from physical threats. This is uncommon but familiarising students with fire exits and any alarm tests that are due during a teaching session will help to alleviate any fear. The more common safety requirements that you need to consider is avoidance of threat to a student's ego. It is therefore important not to intimidate individuals when questioning them. When asking questions leave them open to the whole group rather than singling out an individual.

Social needs

Included in these needs is the sense of belonging and acceptance into a group. As the teacher you can help to facilitate the development of this, below are some suggestions:

- Allow students to socialise for a few minutes prior to starting the session.
- Get students to introduce themselves.
- Organise group activities at the beginning of the session to encourage them to openly share their attitudes and become familiar with one another.
- Organise the seating in a diplomatic manner for small group teaching eg a horse shoe shape.
- In a clinical environment make sure the students are introduced to all the staff members and are familiar with the rules that apply in that environment which can otherwise be very daunting, for example where hand washing/alcohol gel use is expected, be explicit.

Esteem needs

Students need to develop a sense of self-worth, respect and confidence. When teaching in a clinical environment remember that students will be fearful of making a mistake on a real patient. Providing simple simulation environments, particularly for clinical skills, can prove invaluable. We must show concern and interest in our students and be committed to their welfare. We should treat students with the same respect that we expect them to show our patients. We should encourage our students to be candid with us in terms of what they do and do not know, when they are doubtful and when they are confident, and when they need help and when

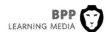

they do not. We should give them permission to identify their needs and weaknesses, and provide a safe environment that allows them to come to us when they are unsure of something, and to admit when mistakes occur. Providing appropriate feedback is essential in fulfilling this need.

Practical points

- When teaching try to give practical and relevant examples for the material being taught. This allows the students to 'justify' learning the material.
- Encourage the internal motivators to learning by asking questions, evoking debate and make the material being taught interesting. An easy way to do this is by including clinical scenarios into your teaching sessions, and asking the students what they think or what they would do, as is often done in problem-based learning teaching.
- Try to understand the different ways in which people learn and use strategies in your teaching sessions that will involve the students. For example, problem-based work in small groups will appeal to pragmatists, activists and theorists. Including a reflective period at the end of the session, where students evaluate what they have learned and identify further learning needs, will be useful for reflective learners.

Key points

- Each learner is an individual and has unique needs.
- Individualise, personalise and give ownership to the adult learner.
- PDPs are a good way to identify learning needs and serve to focus motivation and structure learning.

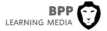

- Having an understanding of learning styles enables you to adapt your teaching to an individual student's preferred method.
- The creation of a safe environment for a student involves considering physiological, safety, social and esteem needs.

References

APTECH Global Learning Solutions. http://leanlearning.wikispaces.com/instructional-design (accessed 05/05/2010)

Bullock I, Davies M, Lockey A and Mackway-Jones. (2nd ed.) (2008) *Pocket Guide to Teaching for Medical Instructors* (Oxford: Blackwell Publishing) pp. 4–5

Entwistle N J (1998) Motivations and Approaches to Studying: Motivating and Conceptions of Teaching, in Thompson G, Armstrong S, Brown S (eds.) *Motivating Students*. (London: Kogan Page) pp. 15–23

Fry H, Ketteridge S, Marshall S A (2nd ed.) (1999) *Handbook for Teaching and Learning in Higher Education: Enhancing Academic Practice* (London: Kogan Page) pp. 68–71 and p. 180

Harvey L (2009). Analytic Quality Glossary. www.qualityresearchinternational.com/glossary/pdp.htm (accessed 05/05/2010)

Honey P and Mumford A (1982) *The Manual of Learning Styles* (Maidenhead: Peter Honey)

Jackson NJ (2001) 'What is PDP?' *LTSN Working Paper 1* (www.heacademy.ac.uk/assets/documents/resources/resourcedatabase/id65_Personal_Development_Planning_what_does_it_mean.rtf)

Knowles M S (1975) *Self-directed Learning: A Guide for Learners and Teachers* (New York: Association Press)

Kolb D A (1984) *Experiential Learning*, Englewood Cliffs (New Jersey: Prentice Hall)

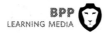

Manlone T W & Lepper M R (1987) 'Making Learning Fun: Taxonomy of Intrinsic Motivations for Learning' in Snow R E & Farr M J (eds.) *Aptitude, Learning and Instruction: III. Cognitive and Affective Process Analyses*. Erlbaum, Hilsdale, NJ

Maslow A (1970) *Motivation and Personality* (New York: Harper and Row)

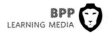

Chapter 4

The skills required of an effective teacher

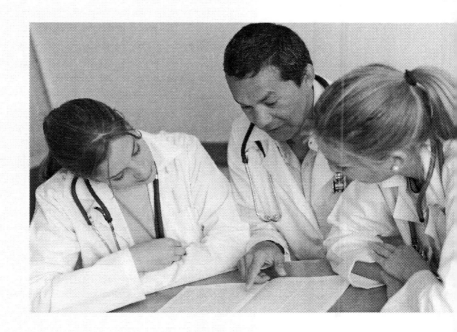

Chapter 4

The skills required of an effective teacher

Introduction

'The greatest difficulty in life is to make knowledge effective, to convert it into practical wisdom'

Sir William Osler

Becoming an effective teacher is a process of continual refinement. As teachers we must leave aside our egos and consider the needs of our students. These needs are paramount if we are to excel in our role as teachers. Through reflection we will develop an individual teaching philosophy alongside our personal priorities and objectives. This is a process that will be in constant flux and must be revisited periodically to facilitate personal growth as a teacher and incorporate new ideas on teaching.

In this chapter we will look at the fundamental qualities that are required to become good teachers and mentors.

 Pause for thought
- List the points that you think are important to be a good teacher.
- Why do you think each of these is important?

Good teachers

There are many things that make good teachers but some of the most important are also the most obvious. Below is a list of some of the qualities required or we need to develop in order to be a good teacher:

- **A command of the content to be taught** – you must understand the material that you are teaching. A superficial understanding will only perpetuate superficial learning. If deep learning is our goal then a detailed understanding is a pre-requisite.
- **Good at explaining things** – this is essential if we wish our students to have an understanding of medicine.

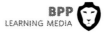

- **Detail oriented** – this goes hand in hand with the aforementioned skills and is essential to trigger deep learning and understanding of material.
- **Common sense** – this is perhaps the most useful skill a doctor can have. Detailed factual knowledge, deep understanding and common sense are the most potent weapons in the arsenal of any doctor and the demonstration of common sense medicine begins with teachers.
- **A sense of humour** – this is an important life skill as well as a good teaching skill. It helps to break down barriers between teacher and student and create an environment that is friendly and open to learning. However, humour should be used sparingly!
- **Fair-minded** – teachers need to be able to assess students on their ability and performance, not on the students' personal qualities.
- **Able to remain calm** – at times we will all be challenged. We must learn to control our urges to shout and scream. Learning about posture, and how to use our tone of voice, and other non-verbal communication skills can help a teacher to assert authority while remaining calm and avoiding shouting.
- **Can manage time effectively** – this is absolutely essential. Not only in the classroom where there are time restraints, but when preparing teaching sessions it is important to manage your time well. This is also an essential requirement when planning teaching sessions. The best teachers plan each session allowing time for questions, demonstrations etc.
- **Enthusiastic** – we can all remember those teachers who always seemed like they wanted to be somewhere else! They made us feel like we wanted to be somewhere else too! If you are not enthusiastic about both teaching and your subject matter then this will come across to the students. They in turn will not feel engaged and a downward spiral will ensue. If you have options about what you can teach always try to teach something you find enjoyable. This will be of benefit to both the teacher and the student.
- **Good role models** – it is important to be congruent in what you say and how you act, for example if you tell your students to begin every cardiovascular examination by observing from the end of the bed but in reality start by listening to the heart, the students will be confused. They are more likely to

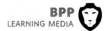

do what they **see** you doing rather than what you **say** they should do.

Many, if not all, teachers do not begin their teaching careers having all the qualities listed above. As with other areas we must work to improve our knowledge and understanding of teaching to become better teachers.

 Pause for thought
Why do you teach?

See one, do one, teach one

Many teachers teach in the same manner that they were taught. They may refine their teaching methods to some degree but overall they stick to what they know. Obviously if they were subject to very good teaching then this may not be such a bad thing, but if their teaching was poor they may unwittingly continue a cycle of poor practice. As stated at the beginning of the chapter, introspection and reflection are essential to becoming a good teacher – teachers must really want to teach and enjoy teaching. Anyone can be a bad teacher but to be a great teacher takes effort!

The age-old adage in medicine is 'see one, do one, teach one'. In certain respects this is very useful. It encourages the student to be actively involved very quickly and to start teaching others quickly too. If we take the phrase literally, as many doctors do, it is fraught with problems. A much better approach would be:

- **See lots of the same thing performed by different people** – when learning skills it is best to watch many people perform the same task since different people have different ways of doing things.
- **Do lots under supervision and then independently** – the only way to become confident is to perform the task repeatedly. You will encounter difficulties that you will need to resolve, (sometimes with help) and develop your own reasoning for doing things. Doing the procedures under supervision will

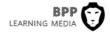

provide the early safety net and guidance to perfect your technique. Independent performance will build confidence.

- **Teach anyone and everyone you can** – now you can teach the procedure effectively. After you have developed your own technique you should be able to explain how and why you do things in a particular way. This will then help your students to become proficient in performing the task and your confidence will be demonstrated to your students. Teaching lots of people will help improve your teaching ability.

Although this does not have the same ring to it, it is a much more logical way to both learn and teach. Importantly it encourages the teacher to think about why they do something and to impart this knowledge to their students. If someone is given a valid reason for doing something they are much more likely to do it than if they are simply told 'this is how it has always been done'!

This way of thinking also extends to theoretical teaching. It is relatively easy to put together a short presentation and then use a standard lecture format to teach a group of students. What is more difficult is to get the students thinking, interacting and questioning but this is how deep learning occurs.

 Pause for thought
In your next teaching session think about how and why you are using a particular method of teaching – is it best for your students or for you?

Teaching models

There are many different teaching models but of most practical benefit is to look at how learning styles are related to teaching methods. As discussed in chapter 3 one of the most widely known is the work done by Honey and Mumford (1986). They developed four different learning styles:

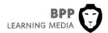

- **Activists** – they involve themselves fully and without bias in new experiences and have the moto 'I will try anything once'. They act before thinking. They enjoy new challenges and experiences but are bored with the longer term consolidation.
- **Reflectors** – they collect data, think about it in detail and stand back before making any firm decisions. They are cautious and consider all possibilities before making a decision.
- **Theorists** – they adapt and integrate observations into complex but logically sound theories. They will approach problems logically and think through things in a step-wise fashion.
- **Pragmatists** – are keen on trying out new ideas, theories and techniques to see if they are of practical benefit in the workplace. They are practical people who enjoy making practical decisions and solving real-life problems.

The above information is not only of benefit for theoretical understanding but can also be put into practice in teaching situations. Groat and Musson (1996) developed a matrix that demonstrated the typical teaching activities that various types of learners would find helpful:

	Graphics	
PRAGMATIST		**ACTIVIST**
Provide demonstrations Provide examples		Provide hints Use graphics to present information about structure
Structure ——————————|——————————— Freedom		
Provide instructions Provide explanations Provide reminders		Provide explanation Provide instructions Use graphics to present information about structure
REFLECTOR	Text	**THEORIST**

Figure 4.1 The learning matrix

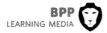

In reality different students will have varying learning styles and so it is often impossible to have individually tailored teaching. However, it is possible to include aspects that each type of learner will find useful into your teaching session. For example, if you have a teaching session around stroke you could start with the theory behind what causes strokes and use diagrams and models to demonstrate. You could use clinical problems to help the students correlate signs and symptoms with neuro-anatomy. This would provide reminders of the basic anatomy and clinical relevance for reflectors and the clinical application would be good for pragmatists etc. These sorts of session involve all the students and engage them, which makes these types of teaching session very effective.

Providing feedback

An important and essential part of teaching and learning is feedback. In the General Medical Council's *Tomorrow's Doctors* the following is stated:

> *Students must receive regular, structured and constructive appraisal from their teachers during the mainly clinical years of the curriculum. This allows the medical school to judge their clinical knowledge and the competence against the principles set out in Good Medical Practice. It provides students with information about their progress and the performance, allowing them to deal with any areas of concern. This will also help the students prepare for the regular appraisal of their performance that will take place once they are qualified.*

As mentioned it is important for students to receive feedback as they will be appraised throughout their careers. Feedback can be performed in a variety of ways, some positive and some negative and so learning how to give feedback is an important skill.

The purpose of feedback is to identify areas where the learner could improve through adjustments. It should be *constructive* and if it is task oriented it should be provided as soon as possible after the task has been performed to allow the student to assimilate the information and make the necessary adjustments. This sort of approach can be considered as regular or ongoing feedback – brief sessions that occur frequently and with respect to regular

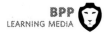

work activities. In addition to this sort of feedback there is a more formal type of feedback given in the middle of the course. This sort of feedback occurs at a postgraduate level and is part of the role of consultant trainers. These sessions tend to last 30 minutes or more, and allow the teacher to address observations made over a longer period of time eg three months. This is also an excellent time for the learner to raise any issues. In this manner the needs of the learner are addressed too.

Pause for thought

List the reasons why you think feedback is important to the learner.

Feedback is important to learners for a variety of reasons: it

- Encourages two-way communication.
- Provides guidance and clarifies expectations and goals.
- Offers insight into actual performance and not simply what the learner thought of their performance. In this respect it can also help reduce performance anxiety and insecurities over performance.
- Reinforces good behaviours and skills and highlights areas for improvement.

When giving feedback there are various elements that will help make it successful.

- Develop a **culture** that encourages and values feedback for both the learners and the teachers. This will go a long way to developing a climate of trust that enables constructive feedback to occur.
- The **location** of the feedback should be held in private and in comfortable surroundings where both the learner and teacher feel comfortable.
- The **timing** of the feedback should be mutually convenient for both parties.
- Performance should be measured against **defined goals and objectives**. These could have been laid down in an initial meeting or be regional/national targets for competency.

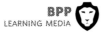

Practical points

Before the feedback session:

- Be aware of what is to be assessed ie if a surgical skill is to be assessed and feedback provided make sure you know which skills will be assessed and how.
- Gather the information you need through direct observation of the trainee. One can and should ask colleagues for their opinions but remember these may be tainted by personality issues etc. Write down your observations and keep an accurate log book.
- Remember to focus on behaviours, which are more easily changed than personalities. Also it is important to remember that people's personalities will clash occasionally but you must remain objective.
- Arrange a convenient time for the feedback and explain what the session will involve.

 Practical points

During the session:

- Ensure the venue is comfortable, secure and private.
- Review the reasons for the meeting.
- Using open-ended questions ask the learner how they feel they are progressing.
- Respond to the learner using the following framework (sandwich model).
  - Start by identifying a positive behaviour and reinforcing this will help ensure these behaviours continue – 'Well done, you correctly identified pulmonary oedema during the physical examination'.

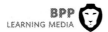

> **Practical points** *continued*
>
> **During** the session:
> - Identify where improvement could be made. You must be specific – 'During your respiratory examination I noted that you did not carry out percussion of the chest'.
> - Give specific advise on how to improve – 'Let me show you how to perform percussion if you are not sure how to do it'.
> - End on a positive if possible – 'The examination skills you demonstrated are good'.
> - Ensure the learner has understood your points and the assessment overall and ask if they have anything to add.
> - At the end of the session put together an action plan and a timeline for the next meeting.

Mentoring

In Greek mythology, Mentor was, in his old age, a friend of Odysseus. When Odysseus left for the Trojan War he placed Mentor in charge of his son, Prince Telemachus, and of his palace. In today's society mentors can be found in all walks of life including medicine. The mentoring relationship should be thought of as a two way process with gains for both the mentor and the mentee.

Why have a mentor?

The specific role of the mentor is actually heavily dependant on the needs of the mentee. This need can vary from helping a junior doctor find his or her feet in the first few weeks of work to helping another, possibly younger, consultant develop into their career.

Morton-Cooper and Palmer (1993) listed the following as potential roles of a mentor:

- Advisor
- Guide/networker
- Resource facilitator

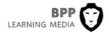

- Coach
- Role model
- Counsellor
- Teacher/sponsor

The role will vary depending on the nature of the relationship.

What attributes make a good mentor?

 Pause for thought

List the qualities you feel it is important for a mentor to possess.

The qualities of a good mentor are not dissimilar to those required to be a good teacher. It is the nature of the relationship that can be different. The most effective mentors allow their mentees to make their **own** career decisions and are available, approachable and good at listening. They should be able to provide both positive and negative feedback in a non-judgemental way and they should help to guide their mentees away from time/career wasting initiatives. As well as helping the mentee with their career they should have an understanding of the mentee as a person so they can refer the mentee for help if they feel out of their depth for example if, the mentee loses a relative or is going through other personal difficulties. The relationship between the mentor and the mentee should be personal and professional. Importantly, the mentor must have a willingness to undertake this role. It is fruitless to force someone to become a mentor if they have no desire to do so. The role of the mentor may also be recognised, through some sort of incentive programme, in order to show appreciation for work that can otherwise be invisible to all except the mentee.

Carruthers (1993) listed the following as desirable qualities in mentors – how does it compare with your own list?

- Role model
- Supportive
- Trusted counsellor

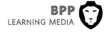

- Good listener
- Interested in the mentee
- Accessible
- Guide
- Experienced in the field he/she is acting as the mentor
- Leader
- Knowledgeable
- Observes confidentiality
- Advisor
- Networker
- Shows mutual respect
- Willingness to mentor

The stages of the mentoring relationship

There are four stages in the mentoring relationship:

1. Initiation phase – the mentor and mentee meet frequently to discuss aims, goals and values. During this time it is important to evaluate whether the personalities coalesce. After this initial phase the relationship becomes more open and relaxed.
2. Cultivation phase – the work begins in earnest during this phase. The ground rules of the relationship are set and the mentee is encouraged to set career goals and list discrete steps in order to achieve these. Over time these goals are reviewed and feedback provided.
3. Separation phase – this can be planned or unplanned. Planned separation gives both the mentor and mentee time to prepare and adapt whereas unplanned separation can result in feelings of anger and depression.
4. Redefining phase – the relationship between mentor and mentee can continue beyond the training period and often the mentee will become a peer.

Being a mentor can be a rewarding experience with some mentors forming lifelong bonds with their mentees.

Teaching philosophy

Developing a teaching philosophy involves introspection and will help identify your personal approaches, objectives and priorities. It

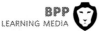

is useful to put this into writing to help you reflect as you develop your teaching style. It is also useful to repeat the exercise to see if your aims and objectives remain the same. It is likely that your goals will change as you develop your skills as a teacher.

 Pause for thought

The following questions are designed to help you write your own teaching philosophy. You can add more information if you feel necessary. Much of the information may be found in this book.

- How does learning take place?
- What elements are required to make a effective learning environment?
- How should teaching facilitate the learning process?
- What is the student's role?
- What are your objectives as a teacher?
- What methods will you employ to achieve your objectives?
- What outcome do you want from your teaching?
- What values do you want to impart to your students?
- How will you determine how successful you are?
- Why is teaching important to you?

After several drafts you should be able to compile a one- or two-sided A4 document that represents your teaching philosophy. This represents your aims and desires as a teacher and will help you to reach that goal.

As well as a teaching philosophy there are other ways to improve as a teacher:

- There are many courses available that aim to teach the fundamentals of teaching.
- Many formal courses such as MA degrees are available including some which can be undertaken on a distance-learning basis.

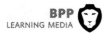

- Learning from experienced teachers and discussing teaching methods with them and your peers.

! Key points

- It is beneficial to take time to think about and appreciate what makes a good teacher.
- An understanding of how learning styles relate to teaching methods can be put into practice in teaching sessions – different teaching methods can be implemented to ensure all learning styles are catered for.
- Feedback is important – it must be constructive, delivered in comfort, appropriately timed and offer clear performance measurement.
- Mentors offer positive and negative feedback in a non-judgemental manner – the relationship is both professional and personal.
- Developing a teaching philosophy will help you identify your personal approaches, objectives and philosophy. It is likely to change as you develop your skills as a teacher.
- Courses and taking time to learn from experienced teachers may also improve your performance as a teacher.

References

Carruthers J (1993) in: Caldwell B J and Carter M A (eds). *The Return of the Mentor* (London: The Falmer Press)

Groat A and Mumford T (1996) Learning Styles: individualising computer based learning environments. *Association for Learning Technology* 3:53–62

Honey P and Mumford A (1986, 2nd rev. ed.) The manual of Learning Styles (Maidenhead: Peter Honey)

Morton-Cooper A and Palmer A (1993). *Mentoring and Preceptorship* (Oxford: Blackwell Science)

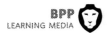

Chapter 5

Fail to prepare, prepare to fail

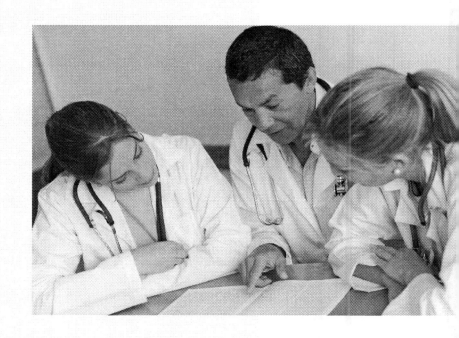

Fail to prepare, prepare to fail

The importance of planning

Teaching can be defined as a *planned* learning activity (Fry, Ketteridge and Marshall 1999). One of the most fundamental aspects of effective teaching is careful planning. Planning provides the teacher and student with clear objectives and structure in which to learn. Furthermore, through planning, a framework is created in which evaluation and reflection can occur.

A plan is important for any teaching episode, be it a ten-minute episode at a patient's bedside or a two-hour lecture. Using a simple tool to plan can be useful especially when planning 'on the go' in a medical environment. One simple approach is to base it on a triad of concepts (Peyton 1998):

1. **Set**: what you need to think about beforehand.
2. **Dialogue**: what happens during the event.
3. **Closure**: how you finish.

Tailoring your approach to your audience

 Pause for thought

- How would you teach a first year medical student to perform a cardiovascular examination?
- How would you change this when teaching a senior doctor who is revising for a postgraduate exam?

Delivering teaching in different manners is essential to meeting the needs of our students and keeping them engaged. Our students learn, achieve and succeed as a result of their inherent learning styles; our willingness to teach them in those modalities plays a pivotal role in their learning. Varying your delivery in longer sessions can significantly increase factual recall in your learners. Furthermore, try to make your students participate in the learning process rather than just listening to a factual lecture as this will increase their retention rates (Fig 5.1) and encourage deep learning (National Training Laboratories).

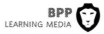

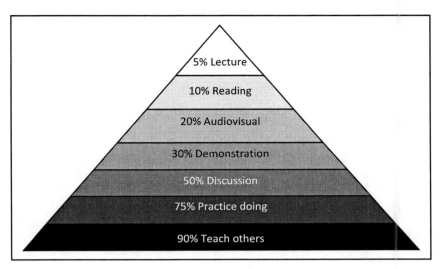

Figure 5.1 Average retention rates for material taught using various methods (adapted from the National Training Laboratories Learning Pyramid)

Being willing to spontaneously adjust a teaching session to the interests, backgrounds, and understandings of students helps you establish a relationship and connection with your students. That relationship is invaluable. It enables conversational interaction, which, in turn, builds trust. In this comfortable environment learners perform at their best. In order to tailor your teaching session and learning materials to your audience you need to have a good understanding of their prior knowledge and skill set. This can be relatively easy when teaching a group of, say, medical students if you do this regularly, but can be more complex with postgraduates or multi-professional groups eg a mixture of nurses, physiotherapists and doctors, or a group of any students which you are not used to. One of the ways in which you can obtain this information is a pre-teaching questionnaire. This can help highlight areas of lack of knowledge, so that you can focus your teaching accordingly.

Lesson planning

When planning your teaching ask yourself the following questions:

- **Who am I teaching?**
  Consider the number of students and their prior knowledge and skills.

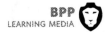

- **What am I teaching them?**
  The aims and objectives of the session.
- **Where will I teach them?**
  How many rooms are available and does this area produce a safe and comfortable environment to learn in? If not how can I improve this prior to the session?
- **How long am I teaching for?**
  Do I need to state how long my teaching session is going to be, or does in it need to fit into a predetermined time because of other commitments? Do I need to provide the students with breaks so they are not overloaded with information?
- **How will I teach them?**
  This includes considering your learning activities and the resources available to you. In this part of your plan you need to decide what type of learning activities you wish to use. Your subject matter will often determine your delivery methods.
- **How will I know that my teaching has been effective?**
  Assessment of students and feedback

There are two frameworks which are utilised to prepare teaching; a scheme of work and a session plan. Both should be produced prior to the delivery of teaching, however if you are simply delivering one teaching session then a session plan is sufficient. A scheme of work is useful when you are delivering a series of teaching sessions to cover a specific curriculum or part of a curriculum. It will help you to plan the teaching in a progressive manner. Remember the Chinese proverb when considering logical progression through tasks, particularly clinical skills teaching:

'I hear – I forget; I see – I remember; I do – I understand'
(Confucious)

You can therefore broadly plan subject matter to be covered in each session when producing a scheme of work.

The session plan is a detailed plan of a specific teaching session, and therefore relates to your scheme of work. It should include more meticulous details such as timings and specific teacher and student activities.

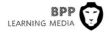

Pause for thought

Develop a session plan for your next teaching session. Think about specific details such as how long you will spend on certain topics, how much time should be spent in discussion, type of feedback, etc.

Producing effective learning materials

Your learning materials have a significant impact on the educational experience your students will have. Therefore it is essential to know how to create effective teaching material.

The essential principals when preparing any kind of learning material can be remembered using the acronym LIGHT (Farrow 2003):

Links – the material you are providing should be strongly linked to your teaching session.

Intelligibility – it should be easy to understand and learn from (diagrams/ flow charts/pictures are usually helpful).

General style – uniformity in the material provided will help focus the learners' attention on content.

Highlighting – emphasise salient points.

Targeting – tailor your approach to your audience.

Presentations and the use of PowerPoint

PowerPoint is probably the commonest learning material used, and many use it to produce handouts of the slides from their presentations. Effective use of PowerPoint is essential. Below are some useful ways of enhancing your PowerPoint presentation:

- Make it memorable (add media or multimedia, demonstrations, video, realism, enable tutor-student interactivity so individuals can respond)
- Use stories, emotions and quotes (eg the patient's journey)

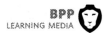

- Only use a maximum of five bullet points on each slide
- Select a good colour contrast between text and background
- Use phrases rather than sentences on the slides
- Use of graphs, pictures and animation to enhance interest and understanding interspersed between slides with text in bullet points

The following should be avoided when using PowerPoint:

- Slide transitions and sound effects (these can act as a distraction and can fail if the computer speed is inadequate)
- Reading from slides
- Heavily text loaded slides
- Standard clipart (this has become a visual cliché)

Remember however, presenting stands or falls on the presenter not the presentation! However, good teaching material in the form of a PowerPoint presentation does help.

Clinical case quizzes

Clinical case quizzes can enliven a teaching session. Case quizzes require the application of information presented earlier in the lecture, thereby expanding on existing concepts and generating class participation and interest in the learners. It therefore encourages the trainees towards the 'deep learner' strategy (Tan 2007).

Curriculum planning

Curriculum comes from the Latin word for racecourse or track. From this it came to mean a study course, and today holds a much broader meaning. Many have the misconception that a curriculum is a list of items that require completion. In fact it has a much broader meaning and it can be defined as:

> *'the sum of all the activities, experiences and learning opportunities for which an institution (such as the Society) or a teacher (such as a faculty member) takes responsibility – either deliberately or by default.'* (Coles 2003)

As discussed in Chapter 2, the curriculum itself has components that interact to complete the full experience a student has (see

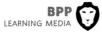

Figure 5.2). This is often a combination of the content that is taught (formal curriculum), that which the students learn from interacting with their learning environment (informal curriculum) and finally the knowledge they gain that the institution did not intend on teaching them (hidden curriculum).

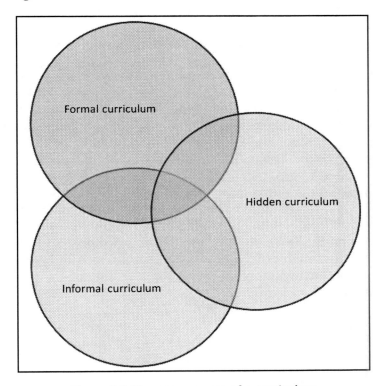

Figure 5.2 The components of a curriculum

Curriculum planning and development are an integral part of medical education and even if we may not design a whole curriculum; as you progress through medical training it would not be unusual for you to have to develop the part of a curriculum that you are involved in.

Described below is a useful ten step method to developing a curriculum (Harden 1986):

1. Identify the needs in relation to desired product
2. What are the learning outcomes?
3. Establish the content to be studied

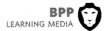

4.   Organise the content
5.   Choose an educational strategy
6.   How will this content be delivered ie teaching methods?
7.   How would you assess your students and ensure that taught content is actually being learned?
8.   Actively communicate the curriculum between those who are learning and those who are delivering the curriculum
9.   Promote an appropriate educational climate in which learning can occur
10. Manage the curriculum you have developed

In the medical field the first two steps with regard to needs and learning outcomes are usually defined by government or institutional guidelines such as The General Medical Council's *Tomorrow's Doctors* document. The content to be studied from these outcomes can be harder to establish and may also be open to interpretation depending on the outcomes you decide to utilise. It is important to note that recently there has been a distinct move away from the process model of teaching, in which emphasis was placed on the learning and teaching process, to a more outcomes-based model. In this more contemporary approach, the curriculum is designed backwards starting at what one proposes the end product or outcome to be.

Traditionally curriculum content was organised in a pre-clinical and clinical manner, and basic science knowledge and clinical medicine were segregated distinctly. The major drawback of this approach was that the knowledge gained from the basic science teaching would often be considered as irrelevant to clinical practice in the eyes of the students and was therefore learnt to pass exams and then forgotten. Harden and Stamper (1999) introduced one of the most popular modern curriculum designs, in the form of the spiral curriculum (Figure 5.3).

The spiral curriculum involves revisiting topics in increasing amounts of complexity and depth as you progress up the spiral. Thus new learning is linked to previous knowledge. Through this process previous knowledge, skills and attitudes are sharpened and new ones are acquired thus increasing competence. The educational strategy employed needs to be considered carefully and the SPICES model is useful in considering these (Figure 5.4) (Harden Snowden and Dunn 1984). In this model each of these

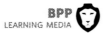

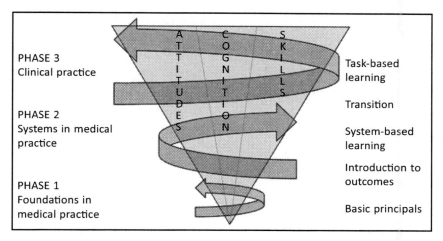

Figure 5.3 A model of the spiral curriculum (adapted from the Dundee Medical School model)

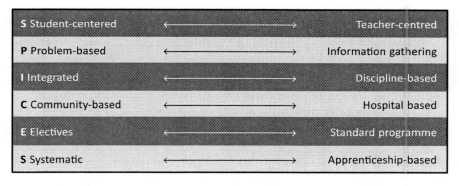

Figure 5.4 The SPICES model (adapted from Harden, Snowden and Dunn, 1984)

themes is a continuum, with more recent developments located to the left, and more traditional strategies to the right.

Most medical schools now teach a great deal of their curriculum through problem-based learning (PBL) or a closely related hybrid incorporating additional methods with PBL at the centre. It is often the preferred method because it is student centred and stimulates students to explore all aspects of a given case; knowledge is therefore integrated and applied. PBL and the other teaching methods available are covered in more detail in Chapter 6. It is important to note however that there is no teaching method that

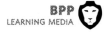

is a panacea for all, and careful matching of teaching method to content and student skill will always be needed.

Assessment

'I believe that teaching without testing is like cooking without tasting.'

Ian Lang (Baron Lang of Monkton)

Assessment can be carried out via a number of methods. Whichever method is selected it is useful to ask yourself:

- Does this assessment measure what was intended to be measured (is it valid)?
- Is it fair (consider the use of more than one assessor)?
- Is it practicable (in terms of assessor cost time and skills)?
- Is it reliable (the same outcome is being assessed on each occasion)?
- Is it acceptable (consider gender and cultural issues)?
- Is it appropriate and relevant to the objectives?
- Is it a useful process for the learners?

Certain aspects of a curriculum are more amenable to a particular type of assessment than others (Table 5.1).

Learning outcome	Method of assessment
Basic science and facts	Multiple choice questions
Clinical skills	Observed structured clinical examination (OSCE) and log books
Treatment of common emergencies	Simulation/moulage and OSCEs
Problem solving/application of integrated knowledge	Moulage, Best of Five or extended matching questions
Communication skills	Simulation with actors
Professionalism and attitudes	Educational supervisors report and portfolio of reflective practice
Ethical and law	Multiple choice questions, OSCEs, simulation with actors

Table 5.1 Outline of learning outcomes and suggested methods of assessment

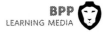

It is imperative that a curriculum evolves with its users; its students, teachers and society. So regular review and adaptation needs to continue once it has been designed and implemented.

Enlisting the aid of modern technology

Modern technology is advancing at an exponential rate. Its potential for use in education is vast and developments in this field have been significant in the last decade. E-learning and webcasting are examples of educational strategies that have become common-place in many institutions, including the clinical education field. More recently interest has moved towards the use of mobile technologies to improve learning eg podcasts and vodcasts.

Wikis and blogs

A wiki is a website that allows easy creation and editing of material by numerous individuals. In a wiki, users can also add links to other sites, and files can be uploaded directly. Wikis are about evolving the same content and improving it eg, students using a wiki to prepare and improve a joint presentation. Blogs are similar but is more like a journal where ongoing discussion and dialogue is displayed in reverse chronological order. These user friendly media can have a number of roles but most commonly prove invaluable in virtual collaboration when working on a project. One can create virtual journal clubs. Health related versions can also be used to educate the public, and for patients to share their experiences. From an educational perspective these tools are excellent as they allow learners to contribute to their construction of knowledge. Most university and hospital information technology departments will be able to assist you in setting up a wiki and blog if you wish to use them as an educational tool.

Podcasts and vodcasts

A podcast is an audio file (usually MP3 format) that can be downloaded to a portable computer device. Downloadable files that are in video format are called vodcasts. This technology is used widely in the music, media and entertainment world. Its progression into use for formal education appears promising. Podcasts and vodcasts are already being used in medical education settings, and their ease of production and use mean that developments

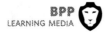

are very rapid. The advantages of podcasts that are propagating their success are:

- Portable, flexible
- Learning on the go
- Appeal to different styles of learner
- Appeal to the 'net generation'
- Selective replay to consolidate particular weaknesses
- Language clarification for non-native speakers
- Empower students to manage their own time (encouraging self directed learning)
- Isolated hospitals/clinics can use them in continued professional development and training

Interactive whiteboards

A normal projector is used to display an image on a specialised interactive whiteboard that is fitted with sensors. This image can then be added to and adapted by the teachers and learners using specialised pens. At the end of the teaching session this image can be printed and distributed to all the learners. It is in essence a combination of a flipchart and PowerPoint. Its obvious use is to encourage students to interact and develop their ideas through working together. In a medical environment one can perceive that it would be particularly useful in PBL. However price and compatibility with current computer systems restrict its use at present.

Audience Response Systems (ARS)

ARS are being utilised to try to increase interactivity between students and teachers in a traditional didactic lecture environment. It is a well known fact that lectures in which students remain passive participants yield low retention rates and hence this technology can help to counter this. It is essentially the use of a handheld compact wireless device by each student in the lecture room to convey their answers to questions that the lecturer formulates and poses (usually on a PowerPoint slide). Each anonymous response is recorded by the system and displayed on a slide as a graph with voting percentages and the correct answer is usually highlighted. The technology has become cheaper in recent years and some medical schools and deaneries across the UK are utilising it in their training sessions. The system has several advantages:

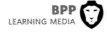

- It can be adapted to be used at the beginning of a lecture to establish what your students already know and therefore focus the lecture you are going to deliver.
- It will encourage participation in those students unwilling to express their opinions in a large lecture environment as it can be intimidating.
- You can assess understanding and knowledge after delivering a lecture.
- You can use it to record feedback.

In a field such as medical education where there are many traditional established teaching techniques, it is easy to dismiss the use of technology as another fashion trend. However, technology can be a powerful tool to complement traditional learning methods. The current generation of undergraduates has never known a time without mobile phones and MP3 players, and will automatically embrace these advances. It is essential that we as postgraduate learners and educators embrace this technology too.

Practical points

- When developing a teaching plan remember that it is only pertinent to that class. The same plan cannot be used for a first year undergraduate compared to a finalist as the needs of the learners are different.
- In the clinical setting part of what is taught in the 'hidden curriculum' is bedside manner. You must behave in a manner towards your patient that is respectful and professional as seeing this interaction and behaviour pattern is much more influential than stating ' behave in a professional manner towards your patients'. Students will copy your behviours!

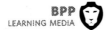

Practical points *continued*

- When teaching use a 'mini spiral curriculum' – always reiterate previously taught material. This reinforces previously taught material but always activates the correct schema and thought processes for the current teaching session. In addition students may also ask questions about previously taught material at this point.
- If there is a large amount of material to be covered think about producing a podcast that will include any material that could not be discussed in the actual session. The students should be advised to bring a portable USB hard-drive and they can download the podcast at the end of the teaching session.
- Provide relevant website details where further information can be obtained.

Key points

- One of the most fundamental aspects of effective teaching is careful planning.
- Take the time to find out the knowledge your students already have.
- Vary your approach to keep your audience engaged.
- Stay flexible and adaptable during your teaching.
- Learning materials are an integral part to your teaching – take time to produce these.
- Interactive learning materials enhance student experiences – use modern technology when available.

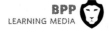

References

http://www.qualityresearchinternational.com/glossary/curriculum.htm (accessed 05/05/2010)

Cantillon P (2003) ABC of Teaching and Learning in Medicine: Teaching Large Groups, *BMJ*. 326: 437–440

Coles C (2003) 'The Development of a Curriculum for Spinal Surgeons', Observations following the Second Spine Course of the Spinal Society of Europe Barcelona 16th–19th September 2003

Farrow R (2003) 'ABC of Learning and Teaching in Medicine: Creating Teaching Materials, *BMJ*. 326: 921–3

Fry H, Ketteridge S, Marshall S A (2nd ed.) (1999) *Handbook for Teaching and Learning in Higher Education: Enhancing Academic Practice* (London: Kogan Page) pp. 41–57

Harden R M (1986) Ten Questions to Ask Yourself when Planning a Course or a Curriculum, *Medical Education* 20: 356–365

Harden R M and Stamper N (1999) What is a Spiral Curriculum? *Medical Teacher* 21(2): 141–143

Harden R M, Snowden S, Dunn W R (1984) Some Educational Strategies in Curriculum Development: the SPICES Model, *Medical Education* 18: 284–297

National Training Laboratories, Bethel, Maine USA. (www.bioscience.heacademy.ac.uk/journal/vol3/beej-3-5.aspx)

Peyton J W R (1998) *Teaching and Learning in Medical Practice* (Rickmansworth: Manticore Europe Limited) pp. 193–207

Tan K B (2007) Short Clinical Case Quizzes: A Useful Tool to Help Enhance Lectures, *Medical Educaction Online* [serial online] 2007; 12 (http://www.med-ed-online.org (accessed 05/05/2010))

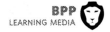

Chapter 6
Teaching effectively to your audience

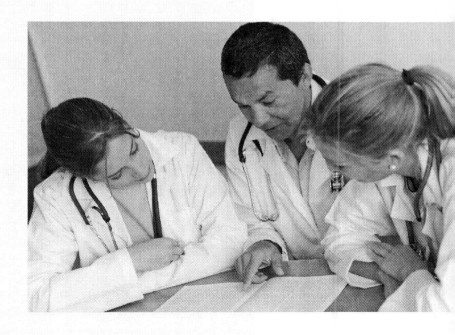

Chapter 6

Teaching effectively to your audience

Introduction

We can all remember great teachers. They inspire us and always manage get the best out of their students. What is it that makes one teacher better than another? Are they innately better at teaching or have they learned and perfected skills that enable them to excel? In this chapter we will look at the different types of teaching and consider the pros and cons of each.

Pause for thought

- Write down the names of your three best teachers. They could be friends, family members, secondary school teachers or even university professors.
- Under each of their names decide on the five most important things that you thought enabled these people to be great teachers.
- Try to identify similarities.
- Did they all teach in the same manner?
- Keep this list, we will return to it below.

One skill that effective teachers possess is the ability to adapt how they teach to the needs of the learner. They feel just as competent delivering a lecture as they do one-on-one teaching. In order to be proficient in adapting your teaching methods a thorough understanding of the different options is required.

Pause for thought

- Try to list as many different methods of teaching as you can eg small group, lectures etc
- Try to think about the number of people you will be teaching – is a lecture to a single person as effective as an informal discussion with a single person? How will the number of people you teach influence the method of teaching you choose?
- Go back to your list of teachers.

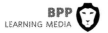

As medical educators we must be aware of the various settings in which teaching is conducted. Some settings are listed below.

- One-to-one teaching
- Small group teaching
- Problem-based teaching
- Lecture-based teaching
- Peer teaching
- Clinical skills teaching
- Non-clinical skills teaching

Many of these different teaching settings will be familiar and each has its advantages and disadvantages, both for the students and for teachers. Understanding when and where to adopt a particular teaching setting is as important as appreciating the differences between them.

Problem-based learning

What is problem-based learning?

Problem based learning (PML) has gained acceptance as a useful way of teaching and learning in medicine over the last few years. Many undergraduate medical schools now use PBL. Dolmans (1994) described PBL as follows:

> *Faculty objectives are translated into a problem, usually consisting of a set of phenomena in need of some kind of explanation. Students analyse these problems, attempting to understand the underlying principles or processes through small-group discussion. During discussion, questions which remain unanswered are identified. These questions or learning issues serve as a guide for independent and self directed learning.*

This description serves as an excellent starting point when looking at PBL.

Looking at the passage, several important facts about PBL can be determined:

- The faculty defines the problem. These are often common clinical scenarios or case studies.

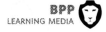

- The students are given the problem at a small group teaching session. This is not a lecture-based method of teaching.
- The students analyse the problem and are given time to consider the problem in the session.
- The problem is discussed. The group determines what the problem is, and discusses how to solve the problem. The students identify learning goals through this process.

The last point is very important. As adult learners we must take increasing ownership of our own learning. This is important not only at medical school but more importantly it is a skill that is required in postgraduate medicine where work and life must be balanced. In determining what is important to learn and what is not the students are learning how to use their time effectively to achieve their learning goals. In addition they will learn where and how to find knowledge – the knowledge is not simply handed to them in a lecture. These are essential skills and it takes time to develop these.

After the problem is discussed and the learning points decided upon at the first meeting the students are given time to devise possible solutions to them. At a follow-up meeting the answers are discussed. The answers are summarised and other areas related to the topic can be discussed to which the new knowledge is relevant. This generalisation of new knowledge is important for students to realise the wider relevance of concepts and principles in clinical medicine.

These are the key features of the PBL process and all the steps are essential for PBL to be an effective way to teach and learn. The overall process has been organised into various different models. The Harvard Medical School Six-Step approach summarises it as follows:

1. The group is given a written problem scenario without the chance to study it beforehand.
2. The students define the problem and/or problems.
3. The group identify the learning goals.
4. Students work independently to meet the learning goals.
5. The group reconvenes and they review what they have learned and whether the learning outcomes have been met. Further

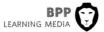

individual work or more group meetings may be required to achieve this.

6.   The group synthesises and summarises their work. The students generalise from the specific problem to other situations.

What is the role of the PBL tutor?

The tutor in a PBL session acts as a facilitator for the learning process rather than the person who imparts knowledge. Think of the role of the tutor as a guide. Some of the effective skills required by a PBL tutor include:

* Maintaining a friendly and open-minded group.
* An ability to analyse the group dynamic and identify those students who may require more help and / or encouragement in expressing their ideas. The reverse is also true to prevent stronger more confident members of the group from dominating the discussion.
* An ability to intervene tactfully but with authority.
* Avoiding direct instruction and simply giving the answers to the students.
* Ability to reflect upon and critically appraise their performance.
* An understanding of the stage of learning of the students and their current knowledge.
* An ability to help place the new knowledge into the correct context within the curriculum at large.

Let us now look at the ways in which we can meet the aims set out above.

Maintaining a friendly and open-minded group will begin before the group even meets. The environment in which the group meets needs to be comfortable and with as few external distractions as possible eg outside noise etc. Ample comfortable seating is required along with any other equipment, for example projectors, TV screens etc, that you may require. When the group meet for the first time each member should introduce themselves to the other members and the facilitator. The aim of the session(s) should be clearly explained by the facilitator. A brief informal discussion regarding the students' prior experience with PBL and their expectations

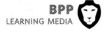

will help the group to gel and create rapport with the facilitator. Trust is an essential prerequisite and an honest discussion of the expectations of the facilitator and the group at an early stage will help to build trust.

The students should sit in a circle with the facilitator at the same level and also part of the circle. This will allow the facilitator to monitor all the students and will help when it comes to feedback/ assessment for the students. If certain students seem to dominate the discussion, the facilitator should openly encourage other members to contribute. This could include posing direct questions to other members of the group. Vice versa, quieter members need to be encouraged to speak without fear of reprisal from either the other students or from the facilitator. It is important to remember that this is the time when all comments should be heard and discussed. It is better to make a mistake at this point than later when it may have serious consequences! Hence, all comments should be heard and discussed in order that all the students understand and correctly integrate the knowledge.

At times the facilitator may need to intervene. This may be required when the students are focusing too much on trivial points and details rather than the overall problem. In these situations the facilitator should try to get the group back in the right direction. Often this can be best achieved by directly posing a question to a member of the group. The tone should be authoritative and the question clear and easily understood. This should only be done if the group is not progressing through the problem at a reasonable pace of their own accord. Another technique can be to shift the focus of the discussion. For example if the students are discussing the clinical presentation of the disease for too long you can pose a question about how the disease is investigated. Furthermore, some groups or students, especially those unfamiliar or uncomfortable with PBL may try to extract the answer from the facilitator. The unwary facilitator will often fall prey to these tactics. Simply handing the information to the students is counter-productive as the purpose of PBL is to encourage the students to think, probe and discover the answers for themselves. Through this process they achieve deep learning and greater understanding. In these scenarios the question can be re-directed to the group or even to the individual who asked the question. A useful technique to

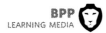

help them answer the question is to start at the basic sciences and builds up from there. For example if a student asks a question about why the pain of appendicitis moves, the facilitator could ask an initial question to the group about how the gut is divided (into foregut, midgut and hindgut) and its innervation (each has a different innervation). The next set of questions could relate to the innervation of the peritoneum, and so on, until the students have worked out the answer from basic principles. Thus the students arrive at the answer but have to work it out for themselves. To achieve this the faciliatator must be aware what the stage of training of the group is – ie the knowledge of first year clinical students would be considerably less than final year students. This will also help the facilitator judge when the new knowledge is relevant to other clinical scenarios and problems that the students can be expected to know about.

The role of the PBL tutor is markedly different from that of a standard lecturer. A different set of qualities and skills is required to be an effective PBL tutor and not all people find this task easy.

 Pause for thought

You are asked to be a PBL tutor.

- How would you go about planning and preparing for this role?
- Will you prepare any supplemental materials eg journal articles for the students etc.?
- What do you think you would need to do before and after the PBL session?
- How will you evaluate your performance?
- How will you evaluate the performance of the students?

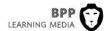

Practical points

After answering the questions above you should come to realise that an effective and well organised PBL tutor needs time to prepare and an enthusiasm to teach and be involved with students. Practical points to aid the new PBL tutor include:

- Observe PBL session(s) in practice before participating.
- Find out if your students have participated in PBL sessions in the past or if they are new to this method of teaching.
- Review the scenario, the stage of training of the students and the goals of the PBL session.
- Review your departmental policy on student and tutor assessment eg self-assessment questionnaire forms.
- Review how students in difficulty can get support.

What makes a good problem?

Since the problem represents the essential pre-requisite for learning in PBL it is fundamental that it will allow the students to meet the learning objectives determined by the faculty. This means that a great deal of thought needs to be given when constructing problems. Dolmans *et al.* (1997) identified seven criteria for effective problem design:

1. The learning outcomes that are likely to be determined by the students should meet the learning objectives set by the faculty.
2. The problem should be in the correct phase of the curriculum and the problem should allow the students to build on prior knowledge and understanding.
3. The problem should be relevant to their future clinical life.
4. The problem should encourage the integration of basic science into the clinical concept. This allows higher order thinking and deep learning, as opposed to rote memorisation, to occur.

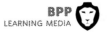

5. The problem should contain cues to guide the students in their learning and in the small group discussions.
6. The problem should be open ended enough to allow discussion and exploration.
7. The problem should encourage activity by the students eg library searches, discussion with clinicians and/or patients etc.

For example, if we consider final year medical students on an attachment in obstetrics and gynaecology, a common real life clinical scenario faced by junior doctors could revolve around a pregnant lady with acute shortness of breath. A poorly designed problem may look something like this:

> A 30-week pregnant lady attends the obstetric clinic and says she has been acutely short of breath. Discuss.

This is too open-ended and the students are not provided with enough information to focus their searches and learning. Discussion within the group could thus become chaotic because of the myriad avenues in which this problem could expand. A much better way to present the problem would be:

> A 30-week pregnant lady attends the obstetric clinic with a history of acute shortness of breath and pleuritic chest pain. She also notes that her left calf has become larger than the right calf. What potential diagnosis are you concerned about and how should she be investigated?

With this clinical scenario the likely diagnosis (pulmonary embolus) is not in question. Moreover the student is coerced into considering the various methods for diagnosing pulmonary embolus. Through their research they will see that both computed tomography pulmonary angiography (CTPA) and nuclear medicine ventilation/perfusion (V/Q) scanning involve radiation, which may be harmful to the baby and the mother. They can appreciate the concept of risk versus benefit. They will learn the advantages and disadvantages of the different methods for investigating pulmonary embolus which will be useful to their role as junior doctors. The problem is still open-ended enough to allow debate and discussion of how pulmonary embolus in pregnancy should be investigated, but it has a finite end-point.

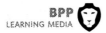

Chapter 6

What are the advantages and disadvantages of PBL?

With all teaching methods there are pros and cons and PBL is no different. The role of the tutor is to identify which teaching method is best suited to the needs of the students and which is most able to meet the faculty requirements. Some of the advantages and disadvantages of a PBL may seem obvious while others may not.

Let us look at some of the advantages and disadvantages offered by PBL.

Advantages

- It is an excellent way to integrate knowledge gained in other parts of the curriculum. The PBL sessions can act to focus and consolidate basic principles. Since PBL helps with a constructivist approach to learning (new knowledge is built onto existing knowledge) it helps the student develop a personal schema for the organisation and retrieval of knowledge.
- It encourages deep learning as opposed to superficial rote memorisation. As students can be challenged by their peers and tutors in the sessions they are forced to understand as well as memorise information.
- The learning is relevant to common clinical scenarios and problems that the students will face on the wards, in clinics and in everyday life as doctors.
- It encourages the student to take more responsibility for their own learning. This is important if the students are to become life-long learners.

Disadvantages

- It can be very time intensive for both the medical students and the tutors. This is especially true if the tutors are moving from a more traditional lecture-based course towards a more integrated curriculum.
- It tutors require training and a different skill set to those of standard lecturers. This can mean it is difficult for some teachers to 'retrain' to be effective PBL tutors.

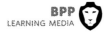

Practical points

- Use PBL sessions to integrate knowledge that the students may have gained from other small group teaching lectures etc. For example, if the students are receiving lectures about cardiology try to arrange your PBL sessions to reflect this. This will then make the learning more relevant and aid deep learning.
- Patients or actors can articulate a real-life problem and can help solidify learning by allowing the learners to 'hang' their knowledge onto a real situation. It also allows the direct visualisation of history taking skills, practical skills etc.

Exercise

- Write down the top 10 diagnoses that you think final year medical students should have knowledge about for your particular area of expertise.
- Design a problem-based scenario for each one. Answer all of the seven points mentioned above in 'what makes a good problem?' for each diagnosis.

Key points

PBL is an excellent way to teach small groups and introduce them to critical thinking and self-directed learning. From the perspective of the teacher it has both positives and negatives. Many of the negatives revolve around problems with time, training and cost of running the sessions. These issues can be minimised by using PBL as part of a broader curriculum.

- Observe at least one PBL session before acting as a facilitator for your own session. This will give you confidence and an awareness of what is to be expected.

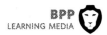

- Spend time planning your problem in detail and try to pre-empt and prepare for any questions the students may have.
- Decided the best way to present your problem – patient history, actor, data interpretation etc. Think about how to make it most relevant, engaging and memorable for the students.
- Decide how many sessions you will need to present and follow up the problem.
- How will the students be assessed and how will you give them feedback?

Lecture-based teaching

Lectures are widely used in teaching with medicine being no exception. Until recently many medical curricula were based solely around lectures and like other teaching methods they have both advantages and disadvantages.

 Pause for thought
- Think back to your own experiences of lectures. Think of one lecture that you thought was very good and one that you thought was poor.
- Reflect on these two experiences and note down what you thought accounted for the differences.

The structure of lectures

Lectures can be structured in different ways. The appropriate way to structure the lecture is dependant upon the type of knowledge or skill you wish to impart. Some of the different structures are outlined below.

- **Classical lectures** – probably the most common type of lecture and the most familiar for medical students. The lecture is divided into broad areas with further subdivision of these broad areas.
- **Iterative lectures** – a type of classical lecture, but with specific reference to medical lectures, various diseases are tackled

 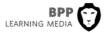

via a common pathway eg symptoms, signs, diagnoses, management etc.

- **Thesis lectures** – similar to a debate, a proposition is put forward and through argument and reasoning it is then proved or disproved.
- **Problem centred lectures** – similar to problem-based learning but on a much larger scale. There is less interaction and more guidance by the teacher and a problem is put forward after which a solution(s) is discussed. A useful way to conduct these lectures is with the aid of an actual patient. The clinical history can be reviewed in front of the students and any relevant clinical findings demonstrated (this may be a video). This requires the consent from the patient. This is especially good for neurological disease with readily demonstrable signs.
- **Sequential lectures** – these follow a pathway from problem/question through to solution in a step-by-step fashion. This can be useful when discussing processes eg physiological or biochemical processes where complicated pathways can be confusing for many.

Lecture preparation

As with many aspects of teaching preparation is essential. When preparing a lecture there are several key steps.

1. The topic – this may or may not be chosen by you.
2. Brainstorm all ideas about your chosen topic and decide which of these you will discuss. Spider diagrams are a useful way to brainstorm and link relevant ideas into sensible groups. Remember that the attention of the students will start to wane after about 20–25 minutes therefore important information should be discussed early and you should try to vary activities or the use of media in the latter part of the lecture to ensure the students' interest is not lost.
3. Decide what sort of lecture you will deliver.
4. Form a title and a rough working structure.
5. Make sure you are familiar with the topic, and read around it if necessary. Acquaint yourself with the needs of your students. Remember that what you think is required knowledge may not actually be what is required!

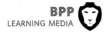
BPP
LEARNING MEDIA

71

6.   Finalise the lecture in terms of what material will be covered, what educational media will be used (eg videos, animations etc) and prepare a summary of the lecture to give to the students. Try to open the lecture in a way that will grab the attention of the students for example a story or personal experience.

7.   Practise giving the lecture in private and to friends or colleagues if possible. A lecture that lasts 45 minutes in private generally lasts about 1 hour when delivered to an audience. Remember to use all media exactly as you plan to use it in the actual lecture.

8.   Reflect on the lecture and modify as necessary. Remember that language and transmission is about eye contact, gestures, tone and pitch of voice etc. These convey your emotions and interest in the subject.

Exercise

Using the guidance above, prepare a lecture on a topic you are comfortable with.

 Key points

- Lectures are a useful way to impart knowledge on a large scale and so are integral to teaching in medicine.
- When used effectively lectures can be a powerful tool in the teacher's arsenal.
- The key to delivering a successful lecture is to prepare it thoroughly and practise it beforehand. This should be done in front of friends or colleagues ideally so they can provide feedback.

Small group teaching

Small group teaching is something of a misnomer because the basis of small group teaching actually has very little to do with the size of the group. For example one educator may find a group of 10 students 'small' whereas others may find a group of 20 'small'.

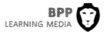

What is important is that the group should demonstrate three characteristics:

1. **Active participation** – the single most important feature. All students should be involved.
2. **A specific task** – there needs to be a well defined task and the work of the group should be focused on that task.
3. **Reflection** – this occurs either at the end of the session or at a separate time. Reflection is important for deep learning.

Small group teaching is important for medical professionals not only because it promotes deep learning but because it also encourages and helps students to learn group skills, effective communication, time management etc. These are all part of the hidden curriculum but are essential skills for any doctor.

 Pause for thought
- Think back to your own experiences of lectures. Think of one lecture that you thought was very good and one that you thought was poor.
- Reflect on these two experiences and note down what you thought accounted for the differences.

Think of as many different small group teaching methods as you can eg problem-based learning, role play etc.

Different types of small group teaching

There are many different ways small group teaching can occur. Broadly speaking they can be divided into clinical (where a patient is involved) and non-clinical.

Non-clinical

- **Tutorial** – the group discusses previously covered material or assignment. The role of the teacher is to focus on the prepared work and after answering the main questions set by the teacher the students should guide the course of the session through new questions, follow-up discussion etc. The

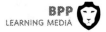

students should be encouraged to answer any questions that arise themselves if possible.

- **Seminar** – the students present a piece of work eg a PowerPoint presentation. All the students should be involved. This type of small group teaching session is aimed at improving presentation skills, research ability, critical appraisal of information etc.
- **Free discussion** – this type of session is designed to encourage debate and the exploration of thoughts, feelings and values. It is particularly useful in the context of medical ethics.
- **Role play** – students take on various roles and participate in a scenario. This is particularly effective in exploring communication skills including exposing students to situations they may not encounter often or that may be particularly difficult. Each person involved will be given a clear role, sometimes with a written script that they can refer back to. The interaction is filmed so that playback can be used to provide constructive feedback.

In addition to viewing the video and providing some self reflection, other students and facilitators can provide feedback using the 'sandwich' technique where constructive criticism is provided in the following order:
- What went well/was good
- What could be improved
- What went well/was good

This is not an exhaustive list of the various different types of small groups session but highlights the great degree of flexibility offered by this teaching method.

Clinical

The most easily recognised form of small group teaching, clinical teaching has been the cornerstone of medical teaching. Clinical teaching is often centred at the bedside or can just as easily be conducted in the outpatient clinic. Clinical teaching will be dealt with in a separate section.

When thinking of small group teaching, including PBL and clinical teaching, it helps to divide it into the Before, During and After.

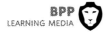

Before

- Determine how many students you want in your group. It is better not to allow the students to choose their own group since this will inevitably result in groups of friends or like-minded individuals coalescing. Strategically choosing a mixed group in terms of gender, ethnicity, age etc will give a much broader experience base to contribute to the debate and learning.
- Ensure the members of staff involved know what is expected of them.
- Identify your objective and determine the most appropriate method of small group teaching.
- Prepare the stimulus material eg handouts, videos, presentations etc.

During

Before discussing what happens during the session it may be useful to review the stages of group development. Tuckman's four stages of group development is one of the best known.

Stage 1: Forming
The individuals attempt to establish their personal identities. Ice-breaking occurs at this stage and strengths and weaknesses are determined.

↓

Stage 2: Storming
Conflict and competition arise in this stage and members may ask to be allocated to a different group.

↓

Stage 3: Norming
The rules of the group and norms of behaviour are established. The group starts to develop its own identity and begins to function as a cohesive unit.

↓

Stage 4: Performing
This occurs after completion of the earlier stages and at this stage the group is performing at peak efficiency with regards to the task. Problems that arise are successfully managed within the group.

It is clear to see that in order for small group teaching to be of maximum benefit the facilitator must successfully guide the group through to Stage 4. How is this achieved?

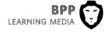

In the first instance the facilitator uses ice-breakers to encourage the students to open up to one another. This can range from a simple 'Hi, my name is…..' to more complicated introductions involving background information on schooling, experiences expectations about the sessions etc.

After this the facilitator will establish 'ground rules'. It is often useful to involve the students when setting ground rules to encourage trust amongst the members. Basic ground rules can include the following:

- All members must contribute
- Only one person speaks at a time
- Humiliation or ridicule of other members is not allowed

These are just some of the more common ground rules.

The facilitator must ensure that the students know what they are doing and the aims of the teaching session. The facilitator should give clear and concise explanations and should also quantify the time available for the session. The facilitator should also help the group move through the four stages of group formation as quickly and smoothly as possible in order for the students to gain the most from the sessions.

Pause for thought

Think back to when you were involved in small group teaching sessions at medical school. Can you recall any instances where you felt basic ground rules such as those listed above were not adhered to?

After

At the end of the session the facilitator must summarise the learning that occurred. This is important because even at this stage misunderstanding can be corrected. Constructive feedback can be given to the group and individuals and students can give feedback to each other.

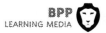

Evaluation of the session is the other key aspect to improving. The easiest method will be verbal feedback from the members through a series of open and closed questions. However, students may feel uneasy at expressing their true opinions and so it is often better to use anonymised feedback forms. This has the added advantage of being a hard copy that can be reviewed over a number of sessions to see if things are changing and improving.

Examples of (closed) questions:

- Did you understand the objectives of the session?
- Did you find it conducive to learning?
- Did you think the group was supportive and encouraging?
- Were the objectives of the session met?

These are examples of closed questions that provide essential information on the overall session. Open questions such as 'What did you like about the session?' provide more detailed information on areas that may require refinement and/or improvement.

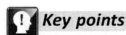 **Key points**

Small group sessions are a flexible way of teaching students both clinical and non-clinical skills. The three main features of small group sessions are:

- Active participation
- Task specificity
- Reflection

Peer-assisted learning

Peer-assisted learning is a very old form of learning and is not exclusive to the medical professions. A simple example is seen between siblings of a similar age – generally the older sibling can help the younger sibling with their studies at school and beyond. Topping (1996) defined PAL as:

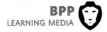

> *people from similar social groupings who are not professional teachers helping each other to learn and learning themselves by teaching.*

This is useful introduction as it emphasises two major points about PAL – the peers are **not** experts or professional teachers and that the tutor also gains from the experience.

There are many different ways in which peer-assisted learning can occur. Some of these include:

- Peer tutoring
- Student mentoring
- Peer assessment
- Teaching assistant schemes
- Peer group learning

The list is virtually endless as is the variation in terminology but in general all these have one thing in common – someone has the role of tutor while the other(s) are the tutees.

The tutors

The first stage of setting up PAL will be to recruit tutors. There are a number of ways in which tutors can be recruited and these have been shown to have varying degrees of success. The tutors can be recruited compulsorily, voluntarily, on the basis of achievement (although not necessarily high achievement), from the same year as their tutees or from higher years.

In order that the tutors feel confident in their abilities they may need time to prepare and do some background reading or prepare a lesson plan. It is essential that the tutors are aware of what is expected of them and in this case clear instructions and possibly even a simulation before the event may be helpful. These points highlight a key strength of PAL that was eluded to earlier – *learning through teaching*. In this manner PAL has the added advantage of helping both tutors and tutees so the overall benefit is greater.

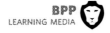

Practical points

- Voluntary recruitment is often the easiest practical way to recruit tutors and it has the added advantage of self-selecting those people most interested in the role.
- Incentives for the tutors include personal development of communication, teaching and organisational skills as well as adding valuable CV points.
- If there is a paucity of voluntary tutors additional incentives such as financial remuneration may be used.

The tutees

In general PAL is open to any and all students who wish to partake in the scheme. In some cases the scheme may be used for the very able students or those considered to be at risk of failure or under-achievement.

10 points to success

Topping (1996) outlined 10 points that need to be considered when developing a PAL programme. Many of these could be readily applied to other teaching applications.

1. Curriculum content – this can be either knowledge and/or skills oriented.
2. Contact constellation – will there be one tutor for a group or will tutors work in pairs (dyads)?
3. Year of study – will the tutors and the tutees be in the same year or different years?
4. Ability – will the tutors and tutees be of the same or differing abilities?
5. Role continuity – will the role of the tutor and tutee be static? This is especially important in cases of same ability tutoring where role reversal can be very useful.
6. Location – where will you have your sessions?
7. Time – when will you have your sessions?

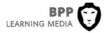

8.   Tutee characteristics – will the sessions be for everyone or will you target specific groups?

9.   Tutor characteristics – remember that the beauty of PAL is that both the tutee and the tutor gain from the experience. Hence tutors with exceptional ability may be under-stimulated by a group of below average students. The key is for both the tutor and the tutee to find some cognitive challenge from the activity.

10. Objectives – decide what your objectives are. They do not have to be intellectual.

Clinical teaching

The aim of clinical teaching is to enable the students acquire the skills and competencies required to succeed in a clinical setting. In order to succeed the student will require an understanding of both basic medical and clinical science.

 Pause for thought

Think back to a clinical teaching session you were involved in and try to answer the following questions:

- Were you directly involved in the interaction with the patient or were you an observer?
- If you were involved eg presenting a history, were you given feedback on your performance by the patient and your teacher in a helpful or unhelpful manner?
- Did your teacher provide information on the disease as a whole or on specific aspects of it?
- Did the teacher explain the role of other clinicians and allied medical professionals in the care of the patient?
- Did the teacher provide practical advice on the care of the patient eg which blood tests to request and why or which radiological investigations to request and why?

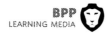

Many teachers teach in the same manner they were taught. In some instances the techniques used are improved and other situations they are not. Clinical teaching is also sometimes thought of as an opportunity to impart more theoretical knowledge with physical, problem solving and interpersonal skills being secondary.

What are the goals of clinical teaching?

It is important to determine the overall goals of any teaching scenario and clinical teaching is no exception. McLeod and Harden (1985) outlined the broad categories that clinical teaching should fulfil as:

- Be able to accumulate and record information about patients.
- Be able to perform a thorough, orderly and complete physical examination.
- Be able to perform clinical skills eg blood pressure, venepuncture, arterial blood gas sampling etc.
- Be able to correctly interpret data such as blood tests, radiological investigations etc.
- Be able to communicate effectively with patients and co-workers.
- Develop an understanding of allied health professionals to provide optimum care for the patient.
- Develop correct attitudes towards patients and allied health professionals.

As you can see clinical teaching is more than the demonstration of salient physical signs!

Where does clinical teaching take place?

Clinical teaching is likely to occur in two settings:

1. Bedside teaching
2. Ambulatory care teaching

In both settings it is important that those involved are aware of their responsibilities. Patients should be asked if they are comfortable having students take histories, perform examinations and practical procedures on them. They should be allowed to decline, but if they

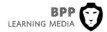

agree, they should be told what to expect and that their feedback is welcome. Students should be informed of the appropriate attire and attitude and be told to introduce themselves to the patients and allied health professionals (nurses, physiotherapists etc) present. The tutors can range from junior doctors to professors, from nurses to senior peers. Whoever they are it is important they have the suitable attributes as they may be (hopefully excellent) role models for students.

Bedside teaching

Bedside teaching will generally occur on the wards. Student numbers should be limited (eg five per patient).

 Practical points

When planning ward-based bedside teaching remember the following:
- Schedule the sessions outside meal times and visiting times.
- Liaise with the nurses to avoid for example drug rounds or physiotherapy sessions. Where possible ask the nurses involved in the care of the patient if they would like to join you. This has the added benefit of demonstrating working relationships and the roles various team members have in patient care.
- Ensure all relevant investigations such as radiographs, blood tests etc are available.
- Secure a side room on the ward for a post ward round discussion.

There are various ways in which bedside teaching can be performed. Some of the most useful methods are outlined below.

- **Shadowing** – shadowing a junior doctor on the unit in which they will be working is a requirement of training in the final year of medical school for all UK graduates. This technique can also be used to demonstrate what the day-to-day life of

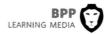

a junior doctor involves. This is a perfect time to be involved in clinical decision-making and gaining experience of basic clinical skills.

- **Teaching ward rounds** – a small number of patients are selected to demonstrate history, clinical findings etc. There are various ways in which teaching ward rounds can be handled:
    - **Demonstrator** – the tutor demonstrates aspects of the history or clinical findings to the students.
    - **Tutor** – each student takes it in turn to elicit a part of the history or examine. The tutor (and potentially the patient) critique the student afterwards.
    - **Observer** – designed for longer cases. The tutor observes from a distance the entire history and/or physical examination and then critiques at the end. Normally a single student or pair of students is allocated to each patient.
    - **Reporter** – the students are not directly observed but are given the time to elicit a history and perform an examination before reporting back to the tutor who is waiting in a side room. Feedback is given at this stage.

 Practical points

Repetition is the key to learning. With this in mind it is often useful to have several patients with similar histories and clinical findings for students, especially junior students. Using the demonstrator model initially, students will **see** how to perform a history/examination. If this is followed by a similar case using the tutor model the students will be able to **practise** what they have learned and watch their colleagues perform the history/examination, and listen to feedback. Hence they will see the same history/examination several times.

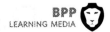

Ambulatory care

Ambulatory care refers to any place patients attend hospital facilities without being admitted as in-patients eg outpatient clinics, A&E department, radiology, day surgery unit etc. Ambulatory care teaching is important because it allows the student to see the patient journey. It demonstrates learning on health education, patient responsibility, continuity of care and resource allocation.

As with ward-based teaching the patients, students and tutors all have obligations. The patients can either be selected on the day, because of interesting histories, problems or clinical examination findings or a bank of patients can be built. These patients will have stable clinical signs and can be reimbursed for their help. This method is often used for post-graduate teaching courses for MRCS, MRCP exams etc.

As with bedside teaching, there are various different ways to conduct teaching in the outpatient department. The different methods revolve around the number of tutors to students:

One student and one tutor

The classical method for teaching in this setting is for the student to sit in with the tutor and observe each case. The tutor discusses the case with the student on an individual basis between patients.

Another method more suitable for more experienced students involves the student working in parallel with the tutor and seeing patients alone. The student then reports back to the tutor. This is known as the Parallel Consultation method.

Multiple students and one tutor

In the Breakout model students initially observe an entire consultation. They then interview and examine the patient in turns in a separate room. In the Supervising model, students see selected patients in separate rooms to the tutor. The tutor then reviews the history and findings with the students in their room. This is a useful method for middle and senior grade students who feel more comfortable with patients. The Report-back model is essentially the same as the parallel consultation method described above. This

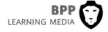

is a good method for senior students as it is most similar to the practice of junior doctors when they attend outpatient clinics.

Multiple students and multiple tutors

In the Shuttle model clinicians run the clinic as normal and they call in students to see interesting patients. The students float between a number of clinicians.

In the Tutor model, one clinician will see patients and keep the clinic running while another will see interesting patients with a student(s) and run a teaching clinic.

 Key points

- Try to keep student groups to a maximum of five.
- Always ensure patients are aware of what to expect with the session and ask their permission.
- Arrange teaching sessions for convenient times whenever possible.
- Involve other members of the team eg nurses etc wherever possible.
- On the wards demonstrate first then observe the students. Repetition is the key to learning.
- In ambulatory care settings the initial step is to determine the ratio of tutors to students. Plan your session to optimise the experience for the students.

References

Crosby J (1997) Association for Medical Education in Europe Study Guide No. 8 *Learning in Small Groups. Medical Teacher* 18(3) 189–202

Dolmans D (1994) 'How Students Learn in a Problem Based Curriculum', Universitaire pers Maastricht.

Dolmans D H J M, Snellen-Balendong H, Wolfhagen I H A P, Van Der Vleuten C P M (1997) 'Seven Principles of Effective Case Design for a Problem-based Curriculum', *Medical Teacher* 19; 185–189

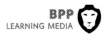

McLeod P J, Harden R M, (1985) 'Clinical Teaching Strategies for Physicians', *Medical Teacher* 7, 2, 173–189.

Topping K J (1996) 'The Effectiveness of Peer Tutoring in Further and Higher Education: A Typology and Review of the Literature', *Higher Education* 32: 321–345

Tuckman B (1965) Developmental Sequence in Small Groups, *Psychological Bulletin* 54: 229–249

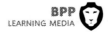

Chapter 7

The importance of feedback

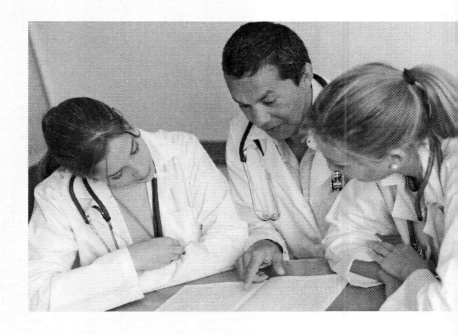

The importance of feedback

Introduction

As clinicians involved with medical education we all work hard on our teaching sessions. For many people it is additional work to their clinical commitment. It is very rewarding, especially when we have managed to inspire and teach students on a particular topic. However, we need appropriate feedback to ensure that our efforts have been successful.

 Pause for thought

Think of a recent teaching session you gave:
- Did it go well?
- What did you think the students thought of it and why?
- How could you make it better for next time?

The above questions are difficult and almost impossible to answer without structured feedback.

Think of a recent learning episode where you were the learner:
- Was it useful?
- Could it have been improved?
- Did the teacher ask for feedback?
- Did you provide any feedback?

What is feedback?

In medical education 'feedback' refers to information about how successfully something has been or is being done, and is provided to help individuals improve their performance. Providing feedback means letting teachers know, in a timely and ongoing way, how they are performing.

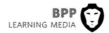

Why request feedback?

Medical knowledge is evolving at a fast pace, along with teaching methods. Teaching sessions, whether lectures, small group tutorials, clinical workshops or web-based e-learning, should be fluid entities able to cope with this. Every time a session is used or taught it should be improved from appropriate feedback. This is the only way to ensure that teaching continues to progress and adapt.

It has been well known for years that:

> *Almost universally, where knowledge of their performance is given to one group and knowledge is effectively withheld or reduced in the case of another group, the former group learns more rapidly, and reaches a higher level of proficiency.*
>
> *. . . the positive effect of F[eedback] I[ntervention] on performance has become one of the most accepted principles in psychology.*

(Ammons, 1956)

Feedback is pivotal to our adaptation of teaching sessions. This importance of the feedback process to the evolution of teaching requires us to have efficient, effective and useful processes.

How to gain useful feedback

There are several forms of feedback. The ideal method is to obtain feedback from several sources in order to achieve the most balanced and reliable opinion. In everyday practice, this ideal is difficult to achieve. However a sound, reliable strategy will help you to achieve good results.

The three main sources of feedback available to part-time medical educators are:

1. Themselves
2. Students
3. Academic colleagues

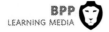

Pause for thought

Think of the last time...

- You were taught – what feedback could you provide the teacher?
- You taught someone – what useful information could have been provided by a colleague observing your session?
- You observed a colleague teaching – what useful information could you have provided them?

The viewpoints from these different sources are extremely diverse. They all have their own strengths and benefits and a combination of all three will result in a reliable, well rounded opinion. Let's not forget that each individual places emphasis on different learning styles and sampling a wide variety of people will allow you to gauge how globally appealing your teaching has been.

There are several feedback methods that can be employed.

Feedback from self

- Checklists and proformas
- Logs and diaries

Feedback from colleagues

- Prior discussion
- Debriefing
- Scrutiny of teaching material
- Direct observation
- In direct observation

Feedback from students

- Structured group discussion
- Questionnaire

Table 7.1 The multiple sources of feedback

Feedback from self

Self reflection is extremely important and not to be underestimated. After all if all else fails at least you would have attended all your teaching sessions! In addition self-reflection can be extremely time efficient as it depends only upon you. As mentioned there are several methods that can be employed. Taking a standard checklist (as displayed below) and scoring yourself on how you performed after each session is useful. Many of these thoughts tend to fade once we re-enter the clinical environment and leave the classroom, thus noting down what successes or failures that occurred and what changes you will make shortly afterwards while the talk is still fresh in your mind can be invaluable.

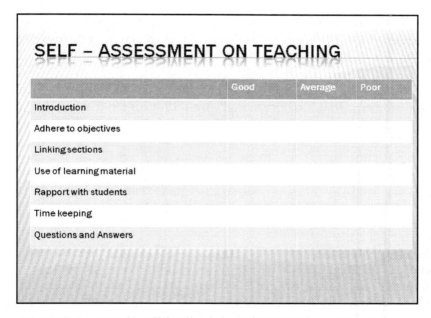

SELF – ASSESSMENT ON TEACHING			
	Good	Average	Poor
Introduction			
Adhere to objectives			
Linking sections			
Use of learning material			
Rapport with students			
Time keeping			
Questions and Answers			

Figure 7.1 A sample self-feedback form (adapted from *Tutoring and Demonstrating: A Handbook* [Chapter 10])

Depending upon how much teaching you engage in you may find it useful to keep a reflective learning log. This could simply be a summary of all your reflective feedback on your teaching sessions. Through time and experience the log will become full of helpful tips and techniques which you could later browse and apply to different situations.

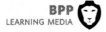

Feedback from colleagues

Direct observation (where a colleague attends the teaching session) and indirect observation (the session is recorded for colleague comments) have had mixed reviews. Many consider them to be inappropriate as they can be intrusive and disturb the teaching session. However, if these problems could be overcome then indirect observation in particular presents a highly accurate method by which a teaching session can be reviewed repeatedly and by different personnel allowing for broad feedback and refinement.

Prior discussion is fairly self-explanatory and involves debating any specific ideas or techniques with academic colleagues in order to learn from their experience and anticipate any problems that may arise. Debriefing allows discussion of the events after they occurred and analysis will allow you to refine your teaching session in the future.

Scrutiny of teaching material is clearly important but it is worth remembering that excellent teaching aids don't necessarily make for an excellent teaching session.

The quality of feedback from colleagues is highly dependent on the openness and supportive attitude they possess. Mentoring relationships are often useful in such instances.

Feedback from students

Questionnaires are a popular feedback tool. Many medical schools employ them routinely so it is appreciable that some students complain of questionnaire overload. It will be better accepted and prove useful if the effort involved in completing it is kept to a minimum. Keep questionnaires short and direct. The concept of the Harvard 'One-Minute Questionnaire' is very interesting.

The Harvard One-Minute Questionnaire involves students responding to a variation of the following two questions:

> 'What was the most important thing you learned during this class?'
> 'What important question remains unanswered?'

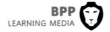

The students return anonymous responses on paper and the teacher can quickly review and respond to these. The feedback that the students receive resulting from the evaluation is very useful as the teacher is able to clarify areas of misunderstanding or non-comprehension that are highlighted. As a result of gathering information using the Harvard One-Minute Questionnaire and thinking about what it means you should have a clearer idea about what your students think was the main point of the teaching and the point(s) they remain unclear about.

Not only is it useful in the immediate setting, it can be used to modify your teaching for future sessions. For example, if a reasonable proportion of the students indicate that the main point of the session was not that which you intended, this tells you that some adjustment to your teaching may be required. Likewise, if a significant proportion of students are unclear on a similar point, or have a similar unanswered question; this enables you to ensure you clarify it in the next lecture or teaching session.

Another quick and effective method is to pass around 'stick-it' notes at the start of the talk asking students to give anonymous feedback. It is similar to the above method but more open-ended. If necessary give them specific instructions to help focus their feedback.

Group discussion is can be a useful approach to getting feedback. The teacher has the advantage of establishing a rapport with the students so future sessions can be tailored to their needs. It is a method by which the teacher can respond to feedback, clarify certain points and encourage debate, in contrast to a questionnaire which is rather unidirectional. However, on a practical note it is time consuming and requires motivated teachers and students.

How to interpret and act upon feedback

The purpose of feedback is to motivate us to refine our teaching. Our response is not only influenced by the quality of our feedback but also the way in which it is interpreted.

The usefullness of feedback depends on circumstance. It has been shown that it is easier to obtain feedback on simple tasks with

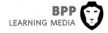

defined and specific outcomes. For more complex tasks simple feedback measures may be ineffective.

The broad consensus of views is that positive feedback is generally more beneficial than negative. However, it is important not to become complacent when receiving positive feedback and continue to work on areas that did not receive it. Negative feedback is thought by some to act as a spur but some are cautious of its long term effects on self-esteem and thus reduced performance. This is obviously influenced by personal attributes such as the teacher's own confidence levels.

Interpretation of feedback is also dependent on its source. Poorly formulated negative feedback from a colleague particularly if senior can have detrimental effects. It is important to be aware of this and choose colleagues who will provide constructive feedback on weaknesses or areas of improvements. Negative feedback from self is seen to be highly motivating. Negative feedback from students can also be highly motivating if taken in the correct manner. It is worth noting though when making responses to the students' feedback: you must either respond positively to the feedback you get – even the most critical, rude, misguided or frankly offensive – or you should ignore it. Any critical, sarcastic, or dismissive response from you whatsoever is highly likely to significantly reduce the quantity and quality of feedback you are likely to receive in the future thereby making your job of responding constructively harder than it would otherwise be.

The more credible the feedback the more effective it is. With this in mind self-generated feedback is thought to be most effective. Feedback from other sources is viewed as more credible when it is based on accurate data and irrefutable evidence.

It is also important to be aware that our own self-esteem influences how we respond to feedback. Studies have shown that, following both positive and negative feedback, individuals with high self-esteem improved their performance more than those with low self-esteem.

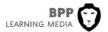

Practical points

- At the end of each teaching session perform a self-assessment exercise as soon as possible and keep a record of your feedback.
- It is useful to have an experienced teacher observe some of your early teaching sessions so they can provide feedback early in your teaching career.
- Perform the Harvard One-Minute evaluation at the end of each teaching session. Correlate the findings of this with your perceptions and use the findings to improve your session before the next teaching session.
- Before providing feedback think about how you would feel if you heard what you intended to say. Your aim as a teacher is to get the best from your students not only for them but also for your patients. Overly critical, harsh or degrading language or mannerisms can have a serious negative impact on students. In addition pay attention to your voice tonality, body language, eye contact etc. as this is just as important as what is being said.

Key points

- Feedback is useful for all clinical teachers.
- Feedback refines learning episodes and ensures they evolve.
- Building a portfolio of reflective learning logs helps identify pearls, pitfalls and personal strengths and weaknesses.
- Feedback from self is extremely important and likely to be the most consistent and easily obtainable feedback during your teaching career.
- It is important to have supportive and constructive feedback from colleagues. Choose them wisely.

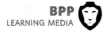

- Student questionnaires are best kept short and focused
- Ensure that you are in the right frame of mind to interpret feedback when asking for it.

References

http://learnweb.harvard.edu/alps/thinking/docs/minute.htm (accessed 25/9/11)

Ammons R (1956) 'Effects of Knowledge of Performance: a Survey and Tentative Theoretical Formulation'. *Journal of General Psychology*, 1956; 54: 279

Forster F, Hounsell D, Thompson S (1995) *Tutoring and Demonstrating: A Handbook*. UCSDA, 1995 (search for 'Tutoring and Demonstrating handbook' on www.ed.ac.uk)

Pritchard R, Jones S, Roth P, Stuebing K, Ekeberg S (1988) 'Effects of Group Feedback, Goal Setting, and Incentives on Organizational Productivity'. *Journal of Applied Psychology* 73: 337–58

Van de Ridder J, Stokking K, McGahie W, Cate O (2008) 'What is Feedback in Clinical Education?' *Medical Education* 42: 189–197

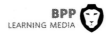

Chapter 8

How to create learning episodes

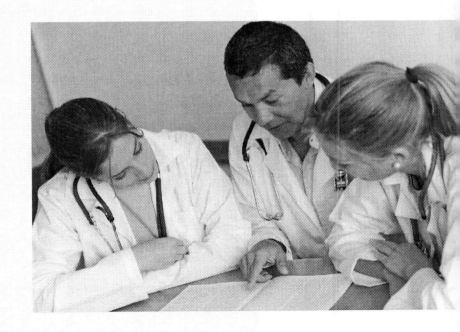

Chapter 8

How to create learning episodes

Introduction

Teaching is sometimes difficult to accommodate in a busy clinical schedule. There are many things that stop us teaching at work. It is not necessarily a priority when we are struggling with a busy clinic, ward round or theatre list. It can be difficult to find time to educate attached students. Some may feel that busy clinical environments that focus on service provision are not a place for teaching. In this chapter we propose to show how each situation can offer multiple teaching opportunities.

The balance between teaching and service provision has always been difficult. New university/medical school curriculums and changes in junior doctor training have led to shorter clinical attachments to individual specialties. This has had a significant impact on the time students are attached to individual medical teams. In previous times students and junior doctors had longer attachments to 'firms' with more opportunity for an apprenticeship style of training to develop.

Shorter attachments have tended to focus training on defined objectives. Students and junior doctors are often required to complete a number of assessments or 'sign offs' to demonstrate various competencies. Lack of confidence in some clinical attachments have encouraged development of workshops and courses to teach students and junior doctors specific clinical skills. While these clearly have their place, there are often many clinical episodes that are not being fully harvested as teaching episodes, where these skills can be learnt.

This chapter presents ways to harness the potential of the busy clinical environment, including the idea of initiating and promoting lifelong learning, essential for all involved within the healthcare profession.

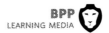

Creating learning episodes

Busy work environments, regardless of their format, are filled with a number and variety of patients which results in a rich environment for learning. An apprenticeship model is an appropriate format to support teaching and learning in the clinical environment.

Before initiating any teaching episode it is important that there is confidence in the student-teacher relationship. It is important for the teacher to have a firm grasp of the capabilities of the student because exposing a student to a learning episode too basic or too advanced for their level can be demoralising for their education and can have a negative effect on motivation. Similarly it is important that students are aware of your capabilities, approachability and availability. A fine balance of supervision while allowing some independence is needed. It is important to emphasise that every student is different and the ability to assess the right balance improves with experience.

Departmental involvement

Students can learn a great deal from just participating within the department. For example getting them to see patients pre-operatively, or in the clinic or ward can be extremely useful. Their knowledge of the patient's history and examination can then be used later on in the patient episode to discuss specific teaching points in more detail.

For example, a student is sent to take a history and examine a diabetic patient presenting for a hernia repair. Later on at the surgery the student can be asked about the relevance of diabetes to the surgical patient. Being armed with a history and examination the student feels more comfortable as he/she has access to first hand information and linking future knowledge to the patient makes it easier to remember and access new knowledge.

In addition, it is helpful to provide specific objectives before the student engages in a particular episode. This provides structure for both student and teacher. Adjusting the complexity and difficulty of teaching objectives is a useful way of adapting similar teaching episodes for students at different stages of learning.

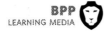

When reviewing the student's findings, raise questions which can be a focus for further learning. Group learning can be promoted by asking students to discuss cases with each other. Asking students to teach their peers is a very effective method of learning.

As part of their education, involvement within a department will teach students about other important characteristics such as team working, time management and professionalism. These are well taught through observation as opposed to more direct methods. But be explicit and suggest that they look for examples of these.

Focused learning moments – specific learning windows

Focused learning moments serve as powerful adjuncts to the clinical learning experience. Short focused learning moments are best employed to emphasise something specific.

Specifically, a student reviews a patient with heart failure. After reviewing the case employ a focused learning moment to review the patient's chest X-ray with the radiologist. This may demonstrate the typical radiological findings of pulmonary oedema. Where possible use of teachers from different specialties allow focused learning moments to be more thorough and memorable.

Focused learning moments can be extremely diverse eg to cover clinical topics, medication, procedures, or to review evidence.

Shadowing

Shadowing is sometimes dismissed as an inappropriate method of gaining valuable routine experience, particularly if unstimulating for the student, or regarded by the person being shadowed as disruptive of their work pattern.

 Pause for thought
- Think back to a stimulating consultant ward round.
- We can easily recollect how much we have learnt from shadowing inspiring characters who became our role models.

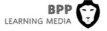

One useful technique is to verbalise our thoughts when being shadowed. It is essential to have gained permission from the patient and have explained to the patient that the student is accompanying you and you will be talking to them about their particular case, and that they should feel included in this. Patients are usually willing to consent. Often the patients themselves have a greater understanding as they witness your explanation. Take care to include them and thank them for their help.

This method is particularly useful in explaining to students how management options are debated and decisions are made.

Repeat, repeat, repeat...

Repetition is the key to learning in the clinical environment. It helps students appreciate the importance of pattern recognition in disease diagnosis as well as appreciate the variety of ways in which patients can present. Experiencing the management of a disease or situation many times encourages self-reflection and follow-up with self-directed learning. It helps to explain this to them.

The effectiveness of complexity

Learning episodes have increasing effectiveness when they are more memorable. Often as clinicians we are tempted to involve students with simpler and more straightforward cases when it may well be the rare complex cases that function as more effective learning material. They create more interest and give rise to more questions, encouraging self-directed learning.

To recount a personal experience: one of the first cases that I remember is a young male patient admitted with cough productive of sputum and respiratory compromise. I doubt I would recollect this case if the diagnosis had not been PCP pneumonia – the first presentation of this patient and with an AIDS defining illness. The complexity of the case and the social factors involved seized my interest and made it immediately memorable. Of course it is important to contrast the complex and rare with the common and simpler diagnoses!

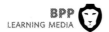

Supporting the learner

It should be remembered, students will function better when they feel comfortable in their learning environment. There are many factors that produce an effective teaching environment, some of which we have already covered.

- Having supportive supervisors and a supportive learning environment.
- Providing feedback to students and getting feedback from students about their experience, at the end and throughout their attachment.
- Having enthusiastic teachers and supervisors who actively engage the learner contributes greatly to a positive experience of learning.

Self motivation

Learning episodes are usually interconnected. One event may trigger multiple learning episodes. Learning may start in the clinical environment but the aim is to continue learning outside the clinical environment. This is even more important with reduced clinical time. In a complex and often busy situation, it is essential that learners take responsibility for their own learning, identifying gaps in knowledge, seeking feedback, and working towards their own objectives.

While students themselves place emphasis on the importance of clinical teaching and the learning environment they feel the key to success is self-motivation, self-direction, and reflection. Therefore, while considering the importance of clinicians striving to create learning episodes we should stop to discuss briefly the role of the teacher in self-directed learning and thus in promoting life long learning.

There are four main principles behind teaching students skills that will help them be continual learners.

Acquiring the skills for learning and practising them

It is the teacher's role to help the students gradually gain these. This is more of a challenge for teaching outside the clinical environment

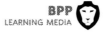

but essentially as teachers we need to 'spoon feed' students less, encourage them come up with their own questions and then guide them to sources of information to find the answers.

Stimulating knowledge-building processes necessary to gain expertise

The knowledge required to deal with a particular scenario may seem obvious to the teacher, but it is often harder to appreciate for the learner. In this situation the teacher can act as a facilitator and guide the process without providing the answers. Much of what we learn comes from clinical scenarios and how we have reflected on it.

Attention to emotional aspects of learning

This includes fostering motivation, as well as helping students to enlarge their tolerance of uncertainty. There are many emotions involved with learning, from enjoyment to feeling threatened. As we have discussed, learning environment and the attitudes of the teams are extremely important. It makes no sense for teachers to tell students that their subject is interesting and important. It is much more effective if teachers show students that learning is worthwhile, even when it is difficult. It is important to harbour characteristics such as taking pleasure in solving a difficult problem and persisting with it. Positive feedback is another way to make students feel learning is worth some effort.

Learning process is a social phenomena

This means teaching social skills and co-operative learning, for example: being able and willing to observe and learn from other people's actions, to ask others for advice and information, to consider others' view points, to relate one's own position to that of others, and to work productively are skills essential to today's doctors. Experience of environments such as multidisciplinary teams and meetings are an excellent introduction to this, and provide much material for discussion and reflection.

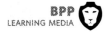

Practical points

- Repetition is an important tool for learning. Even the busiest ward rounds and clinics provide ample repetitive cases and time for learning. After the student has observed several examinations ask them to perform an appropriate clinical examination (after gaining consent). Feedback can be given between patients.
- When there is insufficient time for students to perform full clinical examinations allowing them to experience relevant clinical findings may be enough. For example, a full cardiovascular examination may not be necessary in the patient with aortic regurgitation but hearing the murmur and feeling the pulse are essential. This can be followed up with questions regarding other clinical signs seen with this condition thus encouraging the students to understand the reasons for signs and symptoms.
- Ask the students to make a list of problems for an individual patient under the headings 'acute medical problem', 'chronic medical problems' and 'social problems'. This encourages them to be actively involved in the management and to think about the patient holistically. It is also an excellent way for students to appreciate the complexity of medical care for many patients.

Key points

- Learning in complex, busy clinical environments can be extremely useful and should be an integral and effective part of modern day medical education.
- Using particular techniques can dramatically improve the experience both for us as teachers and for the students.

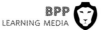

- Specifically in busy environments, it is essential that learners take responsibility for their own learning, identifying gaps in knowledge, seeking feedback, and working towards closing these gaps.

References

Bolhuis S (2003) 'Towards Process-oriented Teaching for Selfdirected Lifelong Learning: a Multidimensional Perspective', *Learning and Instruction* 13: 327–347

Goldman E, Plack M, Roche C, Smith J, Turley C (2009) Learning in a Chaotic Environment, *Journal of Workplace Learning* 21(7): 555–74

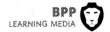

Chapter 9

Why assessment drives learning

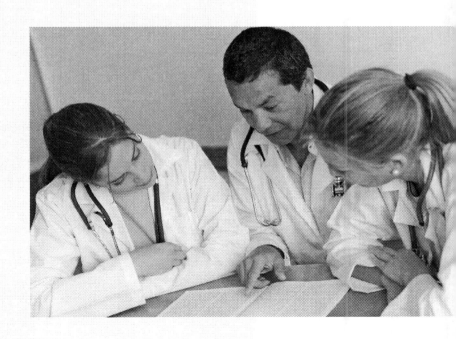

Why assessment drives learning

Introduction

Periodically, medical students disappear into libraries or their rooms to cram for one of the many exams they must pass to qualify. What is assessment and why is it needed? In this chapter we look at the vital role of assessment.

> **Pause for thought**
> - What was the hardest examination you have ever sat?
> - Why was this assessment more difficult than the others?
> - Did you learn more from sitting this exam than others?
> - What was your primary goal for this examination?
> - Was your goal to simply pass the exam or to make you a more proficient medical practitioner?
> - Has the knowledge/skill you gained for the assessment remained with you?
> - Do you think the assessment was fit for purpose?
> - Is there any way in which you think the examination could have been improved?

Why do we need assessments?

Assessments and examinations are necessary milestones in the career of every medical professional. They are an important part of the learning process itself, giving the student a goal to work towards and a time frame within which to work. There are many reasons to undertake assessments. These include to:

- Assess students against certain standards – pass/fail
- Grade or rank students
- Provide feedback to students
- Provide feedback to teachers
- Motivate students

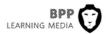

Equally there are many organisations or bodies that set assessments including:

- The government or its delegated authority
- The university and its faculty
- The students themselves
- Postgraduate colleges and societies

Assessments are essential at each stage of medical education. For the undergraduate in the first years of medical school they are needed to confirm progress and demonstrate that students have assimilated the necessary knowledge and skills to move forward in training. At the end of a medical degree the successful completion of a series of assessments results in certification – and the student becomes a doctor. Further assessment allows the junior doctor to receive full registration with the General Medical Council (UK). At all stages assessments act to motivate and provide a source of feedback while allowing the student to demonstrate their progress, by achieving the standard required by the examining body. Students can also sit assessments as part of self-directed learning and educators can look at assessments to confirm that the tuition provided is fit for purpose.

As a result, students perceive assessments as being one of the most important aspects of any course. Early in their medical careers many students focus on passing exams as their primary aim giving little thought as to how this will improve their abilities as a medical practitioner. Once adopted, this approach is frequently continued through undergraduate training. In the past, when there was a dependence on written exams for assessment, junior doctors who may have excelled in examinations sometimes found themselves ill prepared for their first few months on the wards as a hospital doctor.

Assessments must therefore be carefully designed to test all stages and areas of knowledge acquisition, to produce doctors capable of utilising medical knowledge and skills appropriately within a clinical situation. They should assess components of knowledge, skill and attitude.

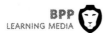

Practical points

You wish to assess a student's knowledge of arterial blood gas analysis. In this situation combining a practical assessment of taking an arterial blood sample and using the blood gas machine with a written station on analysis of the results provides a more 'real world' scenario.

An effective teacher uses assessments to facilitate learning. Effective teaching styles and assessments which are complementary encourage increased participation and avoid frustration. Assessments need to be considered at the same time as course design and curriculum development.

Practical points

Shifting the style or emphasis of teaching to complement an upcoming assessment may encourage student participation and engagement. (Experienced teachers often note that attendance of students at ward rounds is poor the week before an important written test.)

Concepts of assessment and referencing

Assessments are categorised into two sorts: summative and formative.

Summative assessments are the medical school/university examinations where the student needs to demonstrate that they have reached a level of proficiency in order to pass and progress. In summative assessment there is little feedback for the student and the primary aim is to ascertain if the student has performed adequately at the task presented. A summative assessment usually assigns the student a mark or grade. A ranking counterpart to summative assessment is norm-referencing. This ranking system allocates students into a percentile compared to the peers sitting the exam. It says nothing about areas of weakness or strength or about

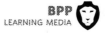

overall competence, only identifying if the student is comparable to others within his cohort.

Formative assessments on the other hand aim to highlight areas of strength and weakness and encourage the student to learn from the assessment process. They rely upon open dialogue between the student and teacher. Formative assessments are usually more qualitative than quantitative with grades and marks potentially detracting from the feedback process. Formative assessments can form parts of revision and reflection as well as ongoing appraisal. The referencing method that most closely aligns to formative assessment is criterion assessment. Here clear objectives are set and the student is graded against predefined ability or competency levels. The student is given feedback on their performance against clear achievement goals as opposed to the ability of other students.

 Pause for thought
- How can summative assessments be modified to yield formative information?
- Are there logistic problems with this and how can they be overcome?

 Practical points

A formative assessment can be conducted at the beginning of a course to determine the baseline knowledge of the students. The students can use this to identify areas they should focus on and repeat assessments can demonstrate whether they have improved. This format allows the student and teacher to monitor performance, encourages dialogue and feedback and helps the student consolidate and retain knowledge.

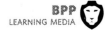

What should be assessed and how should it be assessed?

This question is fundamental in setting an assessment. By determining what it is we desire our students to become competent in, we can outline clear and precise objectives. There should be a distinction between an aim which is a general statement of education intent and an objective which is more structured and explicit. For example the objective 'students must be able to safely obtain an arterial blood gas sample, process it and correctly interpret the results in light of the clinical situation' is much more explicit than the aim of 'arterial blood gas analysis'. Clear objectives aid both the examiner in setting an appropriate assessment testing the core curriculum defined by the faculty and the student who knows precisely what is expected of them. If these assessment measures are established at the beginning of the course students can engage with educators understanding what they are working towards. Competency milestones are an important component of formative assessment giving the student a benchmark of what they should be able to achieve.

 Pause for thought

Outline a core skill you wish your students to acquire.
- Why is it important for them to learn this?
- What theoretical knowledge do they need to know in order to perform this skill?
- What psychomotor skills do they need to possess to perform this task?
- What attributes would you expect them to display?
- Are there any aspects you or others found difficult when learning this skill? Why?

Use this as a framework to outline a curriculum statement for this core skill. You can also use this to plan an assessment of the core skill. Is the assessment a fair test of the core skill? Does it assess all the aspects that you wished the students learn?

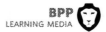

What level of competence is required?

The level of competence deemed acceptable depends on the skill being tested. In some situations a basic knowledge with little practical experience may suffice, an example being students' knowledge of endotracheal intubation and artificial ventilation. In other circumstances complete proficiency may be required. These competency tests are typically to ensure a doctor can practise safely. These assessments are not intended to give information about inter-student variability or produce a normal distribution.

Practical points

- When formulating an assessment, determine what information you as the examiner wish to know.
- Do you need to establish that all your students are highly proficient in a key area or do you wish to establish what range of knowledge and skill exists?

Validity

There are a multitude of assessment tools that can be used, but all tools must be valid, reliable and feasible.

Validity confirms whether an assessment is actually determining what it was intended to. It can be split into five types:

- **Content validity** – is the assessment balanced and representative of the subject matter?
- **Concurrent validity** – does the distribution of scoring of a new test match that of an existing test? Is this test well correlated to another established test?
- **Predictive validity** – primarily used in selection assessments ie admission tests. Does performance in the test correlate well with future performance? For example, do medical students who perform well in selection tests perform well in medical school exams, or make better doctors?
- **Construct validity** – does the assessment behave as you would logically expect it to? For example do experienced

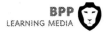

surgeons get higher scores on a laparoscopic simulator than surgical trainees or medical students?

- **Face validity** – does the assessment fairly represent the task it is trying to measure? Techniques that can be employed to increase face validity include the use of models, simulators and actors.

Exam/test formats

Medical assessments are broadly divided into written assessments and performance assessments. When considering Miller's pyramid, written assessments can be seen to test cognitive processes of knowledge and comprehension ('knows' and 'knows how') as opposed to performance assessments which include behavioral assessments (shows how and does). See www.faculty.londondeanery. ac.uk/e-learning/workplace-based assessment/what-is-workplace-based-assessment for an example of Miller's pyramid.

Performance assessments

Performance assessment tools include:

- Objective Structured Clinical Examination (OSCE)
- Short case
- Long case
- Oral examination
- Simulator
- Direct Observation of Practical Skill (DOPS)
- Mini-Clinical Examination (Mini CEX)

The Objective Structured Clinical Examination

The format of an OSCE assessment is one where students perform a series of standardised clinical skills. Each station usually lasts 5–10 minutes but time and station number varies dependant on the complexity of a task being presented. OSCEs usually have 10–20 stations with designated rests in-between, with higher numbers allowing for greater reliability. OSCEs can be designed to assess all parts of clinical practice from basic data interpretation to communication skills and complex patient management skills. In general OSCEs are regarded as having the highest validity and reliability. As a result they are used frequently in summative

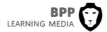

assessments tending to replace traditional short and long cases. They are generally well received by students who feel the assessment is fairer as all students are tested on the same scenarios and marked against the same criteria. They have been shown to have higher inter-rater reliability than short or long cases.

Key basic principles common to OSCE stations include:

- Standardised patients/clinical scenarios
- Explicit and uniform instructions to all candidates
- Manned station with examiner making judgments on clinical and behavioural skills
- Standardised marking scheme with clearly defined marking criteria
- Accurate time-keeping

The examiners and patients are briefed prior to the station and an examiner's questioning of the student upon completion of the task follows a predetermined guideline or script. While it is commonplace for some stations to be unmanned written assessments ie for radiographs or blood test analysis, the OSCE does not provide any benefits over a short answer written test. In these scenarios the OSCE is used primarily for logistical purposes and only provides information for the cognitive component of Miller's pyramid (ie not behaviour or practical skill).

Scoring can take the form of either a checklist (did or did not perform a particular part of the skill correctly), a global rating scale or a combination of both. Checklists are binary where a mark is given if the student performed that individual step in the task. Global rating scales take the form of either behaviourally anchored scales or Likert scales where a judgment is required on the student's performance. They are frequently used to assess students' attitudes towards performing a task ie empathy, interpersonal skills etc. The mark scheme must be concise and familiar to the examiner allowing them to assess the student as the student makes their way through the station without becoming distracted by the marking process itself.

Stations can be modified to increase the level of complexity by changing the candidate instructions. For example the instructions to a first year clinical student may be 'Perform a complete

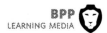

cardiovascular exam on the patient' and for a final year student 'Examine the cardiovascular system of this patient who complains of exertional breathlessness for signs of cardiac failure'. By targeting more specific features on the marking scheme the level of difficulty is increased.

Disadvantages of OSCEs include:

- They are logistically difficult and costly to perform as they require multiple patients and examiners
- They require a large amount of space and access to clinical equipment
- They must be piloted to develop a realistic idea of what can be expected from the students within the time frame allocated.
- Examiners may feel that they are unable to test to depth of knowledge beyond the marking criteria
- They segment history, examination and practical procedures and do not facilitate treating the patient holistically.

Written assessments

Written assessments are primarily used to test knowledge. They are widely used within medical education as they can sample a broad subject area quickly, are cheap to conduct and reproduce. Written assessments can take the form of open-ended questions where students are required to generate the answers or closed questions where one of a choice of options needs to be selected. Open questions are better at assessing a student's ability to use learnt concepts in new situations and apply reasoning. Closed questions are ideally suited to testing factual knowledge.

Closed question formats
Extended matching questions

In an extended matching question (EMQ) all answers are based around one theme, for example cardiovascular examination. A series of descriptions form the questions and the student may choose the most likely condition associated with the signs/symptoms/ test results presented from a given list.

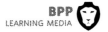

Advantages

Of the types of closed questions, EMQ's are generally thought to better at testing information processing skills as opposed to straightforward factual recall.

Disadvantages

There is an element of cueing as the answer has to be one of the given choices.

Tips for construction

Base all answers around one discreet theme. Cueing can be reduced by keeping the scope of the question narrow, allowing the correct answer to be used more than once and by including statements such as 'none of the above' as possible answers.

True/false questions

The format of these questions involves a stem followed by one or a series of questions that are either true or false.

Example: Appropriate treatment in ST segment elevation myocardial infarction includes:

Tissue Plasminogen Activator (T/F)

Primary Angioplasty (T/F)

Advantages

- They allow large areas of information to be covered in a short period of time
- They are a good test of factual knowledge

Disadvantages

By presenting the answers this form of question is prone to cueing. Questions can be difficult to word and construct, as they have to lend to the answers 'true' or 'false' only. If the answer to a question is false, then no assessment can be made of whether the student knows the true answer. Students may guess if the answer is true/false most of, but not all of the time.

Tips for construction

Recognise that true/false questions are suited to testing broad swathes of knowledge. The test should include numerous short and

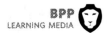

easily comprehensible questions. Try to include as much information as possible in the stem. Avoid terms such as 'always' and 'never' as there are virtually no absolutes in medicine. Avoid vague or semi-quantitative terms such as 'occasionally' or 'might'.

Single best answer questions

This question format involves a stem and a series of possible correct answers, usually four or five options are presented. The student must weigh up the various options and make a judgment about which answer best fits the stem.

Example: Which of the following best describes the tetralogy of Fallot?
- VSD, pulmonary stenosis, right ventricular hypertrophy, over-riding aorta
- VSD, pulmonary stenosis, left ventricular hypertrophy, over-riding aorta
- VSD, pulmonary atresia, left ventricular hypertrophy, over-riding aorta
- VSD, pulmonary atresia, right ventricular hypertrophy, patent ductus arteriosis
- None of the above

Advantages
These questions can test broad areas of knowledge and are less prone to cueing as there are multiple similar options.

Disadvantages
Single best answer questions are lengthy to write.

Tips for construction
Try to write questions where the answer can be derived from the stem prior to seeing the answers. Keep all answers the same length. Avoid including answers that are obviously wrong just for sake of an additional option.

Open-ended questions
Traditional essays have largely been replaced in modern medical assessments with a greater focus being placed on short answer questions and structured essays.

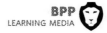

Short answer questions

The format involves a short question that seeks a short concise answer in response.

For example: Which spinal tract does the upper motor neuron travel in?

Advantages
- No cueing.

Disadvantages
- May overemphasise memorisation of facts
- Take longer to answer
- Cannot be marked in an automated manner, and require content experts to mark responses
- Inter-marker variability may be an issue if markers score individual questions

Tips for construction

Make sure that questions are well phrased and that assessors know what is expected in the ideal answer. Give guidance on the appropriate length the answer should be and how many marks are allocated to the question. Only use these questions where others styles are inappropriate.

Assessment, appraisal and evaluation

To most medical personnel the distinction between these three terms is not always clear as they can sometimes be used interchangeably.

The *Guide to Specialist Registrar Training* (sometimes known as the *Gold Guide*) defines assessment as a process 'to measure progress against defined criteria, based on relevant curricula'. This can be seen to closely align with the concept of a summative assessment described earlier. The guide describes appraisal as providing 'a complementary or parallel approach focusing on the trainee and his or her personal and professional needs'. The process will enable educational supervisors to offer trainees 'feedback on performance and assistance in career progression' by means of confidential 'constructive and regular dialogue'.

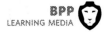

Although similar to a formative assessment, appraisal is usually much broader, stretching past items listed on an assessment form to include topics such as personal progress, career interests, and how the trainee is coping with the workload, study and family life. A good supervisor plays an active and pivotal role in appraisal. They give feedback on performance at work and can act to mentor a trainee through difficult situations and dilemmas, or help them find appropriate support. Appraisal aims to identify any difficulties early, and help to remedy them, with the objective that the trainee will pass their assessment and progress in their career.

Evaluation is usually the trainee's judgement of the programme and trainers. The best trainers and programmes use evaluation to make sure that trainees are happy with the organisation and delivery of their training. Evaluation may be collected anonymously to avoid fear of recrimination if negative. It is also more likely to be honest and useful.

Assisting the trainee in difficulty

Assessments can identify trainees failing to meet academic milestones or having difficulty with clinical work. By combining assessments with appraisal, reasons why a trainee may be having difficulty can be identified, and appropriate support offered. Important principles to remember when dealing with trainees in difficulty include:

- A clear understanding of the individual roles and responsibilities of the trainee, the educational, academic or clinical supervisor, the deanery, university (or overseeing organisation) and regulatory bodies.
- Early identification that a problem exists.
- Establishing the facts and circumstances as quickly and objectively as possible from a variety of appropriate sources.
- Identification of factors contributing to poor performance, which may be work-related, a medical illness or personal problems.
- Identification of the level of risk posed – ie is there a patient safety issue – can they continue to work? Are they a risk to themselves or anyone else?

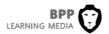

- Appropriate referral based on the level of concern; can this matter be dealt with by the local educational supervisor or does it need to referred elsewhere? (For example to the medical director, the university or deanery, the General Medical Council.) It is advisably to have a low threshold for discussing with another member of the educational faculty in the first instance.
- Appropriate support will be specific to the individual trainee rather than a 'one size fits all' model. This may involve additional training, additional time to allow them to achieve their milestones which may include delay in career progression.

Work-based	Absence from duty; persistent lateness; poor time management, backlog of work; failure to learn and change
Clinical performance	Over- or under-investigating; poor decision-making; poor record keeping; complaints; failure to follow guidelines; missed diagnoses
Psychological/personality	Irritability; unpredictability; forgetfulness; high self-criticism/perfectionist; arrogance; lack of insight/denial; risky/impulsive; insight failure; rejection of constructive criticism; defensiveness; counter-challenge
Social	Isolation; withdrawal; poor personal interactions, including with peers.
Cognitive	Memory problems; poor problem- solving/reasoning; decision-making difficulties; poor concentration/attention; learning problems
Language/cultural	Poor verbal fluency; poor understanding
Career problems	Difficulty with exams; uncertainty about career choice

Table 9.1 Signs of the trainee in difficulty

The signs may manifest in a variety of ways, and Paice (2006) described commonly observed features seen in junior doctors in difficulty.

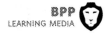

1. The 'disappearing act', where the trainee fails to answer their bleep, is frequently late or often off sick.
2. The 'slow worker', exhibits slowness in doing procedures, clerking patients, dictating letters, and making decisions.
3. Ward rage: displays outbursts of temper and enters into shouting matches when criticised, challenged or under stress.
4. Rigidity: poor tolerance of ambiguity; inability to compromise; has difficulty prioritising.
5. The 'bypass syndrome': other staff in the multidisciplinary team find ways to avoid seeking this doctor's opinion or help.

When one of these patterns is recognised action needs to be taken to investigate further.

Types of training problems

If we can recognise early signs that a trainee may be experiencing difficulties, how do we explore the situation and what are useful next steps?

Clinical problems

These may manifest as a difficulty with certain clinical tasks, missed diagnoses or poor decision-making. If the deficiencies can be narrowed to a specific clinical area, focused training and an extended period of direct clinical supervision is often all that is necessary. An open discussion about what the trainee and supervisor hope to achieve and how each plans to proceed, an 'Educational Agreement', is a useful tool that can provide a framework to work against.

Behavioural problems

These can range from minor disagreements on the wards to criminal behaviour and any intervention must be proportionate to the problem. While sometimes attributed to a particular personality type, behavioral problems frequently manifest when trainees are stressed and feel under pressure. Therefore identifying the surrounding circumstances is essential. In some cases it is useful to obtain feedback from colleagues (here a multisource feedback

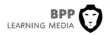

or 360 degree appraisal tool can be very helpful) and guidance or mentoring from a supervisor. Where a clear mal-adaptive behavioural pattern is identified then specific interventions including training in communication skills, conflict management, assertiveness, anger-management and team building may be required.

Health and fitness to practise

Many medical professionals will experience times during their training and subsequent practice where their ability to work is compromised by physical or mental illness. The incidence of depression is high amongst doctors and sufferers may lack insight into the difficulties this may cause. Many doctors feel pressurised to continue working when sick as they think that a period of sick leave will negatively impact on their training or future employability. This belief is particularly prevalent when an individual is suffering from a psychological or psychiatric problem. Where concern exists about a trainee's medical fitness to practice a consultation with the occupational health physician within the hospital is essential to define any limits on practice. The occupational health assessment will also support a doctor back into work after a period of sickness, giving them duties or working hours appropriate for their level of heath. Disability discrimination legislation places an obligation on the employing trust to assist a trainee where possible, in order to allow them to continue working.

Work environment

The working environment and conditions of trainees can have a significant impact on trainee performance, for example, rota design, the level of supervision or support given, or the equipment available for their work. These can be triggers to stress, irritability, poor concentration or a number of other behavioural and health-related difficulties. When exploring an initial concern with a trainee, such contextual factors should always be taken into account. Educators may be unable to resolve such matters directly but should be able to bring them to the attention of an appropriate individual(s) within the trust (eg medical staffing; estates management) or to the relevant Department Head if the issue concerns workload.

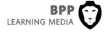

Suggestions on how to intervene

When it is felt that the difficulties a trainee is experiencing are relatively minor and pose no significant threat to patients, colleagues, or the trainee themself, it is appropriate for the trainee's academic or educational supervisor to arrange a meeting and attempt to resolve the problems directly. The trainer should anticipate defensive, guarded or negative responses from trainees and these are only natural.

- Prior to the meeting the educational supervisor should establish the degree of risk involved and determine the appropriate level at which to deal with the problem.
- The supervisor should attempt to attain as much objective information about the issues of concern as possible from staff (via MSFs, records etc).
- The trainee should be invited to a private consolation about the matter/s of concern and a meeting arranged at a time convenient for both trainee and supervisor.
- The meeting should be held in private, and attendance limited to those absolutely necessary (most often just the supervisor, sometimes with a second person such as an human resources adviser). This meeting should not feel like a trial with the trainee as the accused!
- The concerns should be outlined and documented and surrounding circumstances systematically explored.
- The trainee's perspective should be actively sought.
- Desired outcomes should be arrived at after open dialogue with input from both parties. These should be documented. Sometimes it is helpful to remember the acronym 'SMART' (Specific, Measurable, Achievable, Relevant, Time focused).
- An agreed plan of action should be formulated and the actions and responsibilities of both parties acknowledged, documented and signed, with each party receiving a copy.
- Documentation should follow similar guidelines to that of medical note keeping, being legible, accurate, complete and contemporaneous.
- A time frame to achieve the documented goals should be outlined and a follow-up meeting scheduled to review progress.

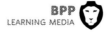

Follow-up meetings

The same format should apply to any follow-up meetings. Successful completion of the agreed action plan should be evidence-based and documented but can include a wide range of sources including work-based assessments, multisource feedbacks or even personal reflections documenting improved satisfaction with work or clearer career goals. If it is felt that the objectives have not been achieved options include a further period of time, if goals can be realised (for example evidence of continuing improvement), or the matter will need to be escalated to the next level of intervention eg the university or deanery.

CPD and revalidation

The topic of revalidation is becoming increasingly relevant to UK doctors as the General Medical Council moves from registration to licensing. Medical practitioners will be required to hold a 'licence to practice', the renewal of which will be governed by a process of revalidation.

Revalidation is designed and needed to demonstrate to the public, patients, employers and colleagues that doctors registered with a licence are fit to practice and their medical knowledge and skills reach the required standards. To achieve this, doctors must demonstrate their ability to practice based on local evaluation of their performance against national standards, both generic and specialty-based, that are approved by the GMC in the UK. This includes continuing professional development (CPD).

The specific requirements of the revalidation process for doctors in the UK are determined by the GMC, and include continuing professional development (CPD).

> *You must keep your knowledge and skills up to date throughout your working life. In particular, you should take part regularly in educational activities which maintain and further develop your competence and performance.*
>
> (*Good Medical Practice*, 2006)

There is no sharp division between continuing medical education and continuing professional development. During the past decade

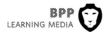

continuing medical education has come to include managerial, social, and personal skills, areas outside traditional clinical medical expertise.

Principles of continuing professional development

- CPD contributes to improved patient healthcare and the overall health of society in a broad context.
- Each individual is responsible for taking part in, and recording, their own relevant CPD activities.
- CPD also helps doctors to improve their professional effectiveness, career opportunities and work satisfaction.

CPD should cover all areas of Good Medical Practice (as defined by the GMC). These are:

1. Good professional practice
2. Maintaining good medical practice
3. Relationships with patients
4. Working with colleagues
5. Teaching and training
6. Probity and health

CPD should include public and patient involvement. For example, representatives of patients and the public may be involved in developing CPD schemes, setting standards and monitoring quality.

Annual appraisal allows doctors to discuss and review their CPD with a peer or manager in a structured way. Appraisal provides a way of making sure that any CPD undertaken is relevant to a doctor's practice and learning needs. A personal development plan should be developed to ensure that a doctor has the skills needed for their practice.

Assessment measures, where available, may be used for part of doctors' CPD. They will help doctors demonstrate their abilities. Currently, valid and reliable assessment tools and systems have not yet been agreed.

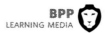

! Key points

- Assessments and examinations assess students against standards, provide them with motivation and can offer feedback for both student and teacher.
- Assessments should facilitate learning and be carefully designed, using clear and precise objectives.
- It is important to be aware of the types of examinations and questions offered in medical assessments as by understanding aspects such as how they are scored, how they may be modified to offer different levels of complexity, and appreciating the advantages and disadvantages of each, effective assessments can be designed.
- Assessments can help identify trainees in difficulty, leading to appropriate support.
- Intervention when a trainee is experiencing difficulty needs to be handled carefully and requires an agreed plan of action, clear time frame and follow-up meetings.
- Revalidation requires doctors to keep their skills up to date and demonstrate their continued fitness to practise. It includes CPD which should cover all areas of Good Medical Practice.

References

'A Reference Guide for Postgraduate Specialty Training in the UK' (http://www.mmc.nhs.uk/pdf/Gold%20Guide%202010%20 Fourth%20Edition%20v08.pdf, accessed 19/9/11)

Good Medical Practice (2006) London: GMC. http://www.gmc-uk. org/static/documents/content/GMP_0910.pdf

Paice E (2006) 'The Role of Education and Training' In: Cox J, King J, Hutchinson A and McAvoy P (eds) *Understanding Doctors' Performance*, pp. 78–90. (Oxford: Radcliffe Publishing)

Further reading

National Association of Clinical Tutors (2008) 'Managing Trainees in Difficulty: Practical Advice for Educational and Clinical Supervisors' (www.nact.org.uk/pdf_documents, accessed 19/9/11)

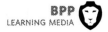

Chapter 10

Use of technology in medical education

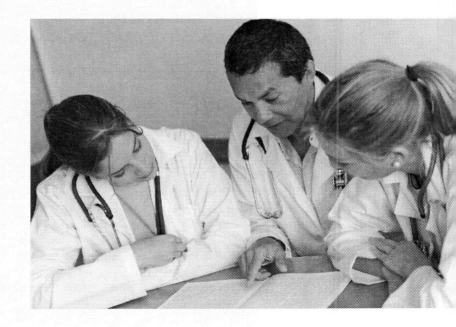

Use of technology in medical education

Introduction

As technology has advanced there has been an emergence of new ways of teaching medical students. From online distance learning to real-time simulators this is a trend that is likely to expand.

From both the patient's perspective, and the teacher and student's perspective it is no longer acceptable to begin learning practical procedures on the patient.

Simulators

Simulation-based medical education allows students to learn from a variety of resources that aim to mimic real life educational and practical situations. These can range from simple, cheap 'low-tech' models to high fidelity computerised simulators that are programmed to respond to the student's actions and mimic real-life events. Simulation can provide a high level of cognitive mapping or learning, when there is a high correlation between what the trainee does in the simulated situation and in real life.

Low-tech simulation modalities

These have been used in medical training for some years. They can be divided into various categories including:

Anatomical tools – three-dimensional anatomical models and cadaveric specimens that allow students to orientate themselves to macroscopic and microscopic anatomical structures.

Conceptual models – these demonstrate simplified physiological principles in ways that are easy to understand and visualise eg a balloon inside a glass jar shows that a change in chest volume and pressure draws air in and out of the lungs. A familiar example is the use of a model pelvis and doll to simulate the progression of the foetus down the birth canal and a variety of presentations.

Procedural models – these allow students to practise and gain confidence in clinical skills that may be difficult, painful or

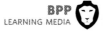

embarrassing to perform on a patient without prior experience. Such models include artificial arms for cannulation and venepuncture, genitourinary models for catheterisation and models designed for breast, vaginal and prostate examination.

Technical models – these models focus more specifically at replicating the 'feel' of medical situations. They include the use of animal tissue for mock surgical practice eg using animal bowel to perform anastamoses. In these scenarios it is important that the model replicates the real life behaviour of tissues involved, rather than using artificial models that look realistic but behave differently.

Simulated and standardised patients – actors and 'expert' patients can be employed for students with limited experience to take a history, discuss a problem or deliver 'bad news' for example in a less pressurised setting. They provide a safe resource for students to learn from their mistakes. Patients can be briefed on how much information to give before prompting thus enabling less experienced trainees to reach a diagnosis even if they have failed to ask all the pertinent questions initially. Patients and actors can give feedback on performance based on their interactions with other trainees/ doctors. If instructed to behave in a standardised manner, simulated patients are an excellent resource for examinations and assessments and are frequently utilised within an OSCE setting.

Practical points

When first introducing a new learning outcome it is usually a good plan to select a single simulation type, and as students progress through their training, combining various strategies can be beneficial. For example having an actor with a simulated laceration attached to his arm allows the trainee to enter into conversation with the patient, enquire about the injury and medical history and provide reassurance and information as they proceed with the treatment. In this scenario the trainee learns to interact with the patient holistically in a situation that more closely mimics real life.

Practical points *continued*

For a student who has no experience of suturing and needs to concentrate all their focus on the procedural task alone it is better for them to gain experience of the practical task first, and then move onto dealing with patient interaction at the same time.

 Pause for thought
- Do you already use simulation in your teaching?
- In what ways can you combine low-tech simulations to produce more 'life-like' situations?
- Are you using simulation to test human factors and non-procedural skills?
- Can you adapt your current methods to incorporate these components?

High-tech simulation

What are the options for using this new technology?

Screen-based simulation

The simplest of these involves the conversion of low-tech models to computer models which can be used to demonstrate anatomical or conceptual processes using computer animation. These can be integrated with other online resources to produce whole educational modules and have been adopted by many medical schools and post-graduate educational bodies. The inclusion of videos with patient histories, diagnostic tests, and surgical procedures and the ability to raise ethical considerations allow students to experience, reflect and learn from all aspects of a patient's journey in an easily accessible format. While costly to produce initially, these tools have a broad scope and can be used by many students if accessible online. There is also the possibility for integrating assessment and feedback thus providing valuable information to students and faculty alike.

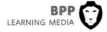 BPP
LEARNING MEDIA

High-fidelity procedural simulation

As well as utilising new software on existing computers, many immersive simulator systems have been developed to accurately simulate complicated medical and surgical procedures. They can be compared to the flight simulators that have been used in the aviation industry for several decades. These devices have been developed to simulate clinical examination skills, such as auscultation; investigative techniques including angiography and ultrasonography; and technical skills such as endoscopic and laparoscopic procedures. Microsurgical simulators have also been developed for specialties such as ophthalmology. These aim to provide a realistic and interactive experience and are therefore ideally suited to tasks where the procedure is normally viewed on screen. Similar technology has been incorporated into simulated microscopes. The controls used to perform the tasks are designed to look, feel and behave like actual instruments with more sophisticated simulators providing tactile feedback as well. The devices come with a catalogue of scenarios and training tasks, which can usually be expanded by software updates. Scenarios can include unanticipated findings and complications and the difficulty of tasks can often be increased as the trainee becomes more familiar and proficient with the use of the simulator. While very versatile, the tasks are frequently preprogrammed with limited scope for a trainer to influence the scenario or outcome. On completion of the task the simulator usually provides data on performance, such as time taken, conservation of motion and correct identification of pathological structures. One should be cautious of placing too high a dependence on these outcome measures, and use as a guide only, as different simulators have been validated to a greater or lesser degree. However, they are useful ways of gaining experience and judging some level of expertise at a procedure.

Interactive patient simulators

The most sophisticated simulators are those that not only replicate tasks but also replicate the environment in which they are performed. High-fidelity simulated patients have been produced and are utilised within dedicated simulation centres. These are designed to look and function like operating theatres or resuscitation rooms. They go beyond a computerised flight simulator and become a whole artificial cockpit. The simulated patients vary in level of

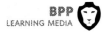

sophistication, with the most advanced allowing the trainer to speak to the trainee/operator as if they were the patient, via a concealed microphone. They have audible breath and heart sounds and produce a selectable ECG trace when attached to a monitor. The models can be cannulated, intubated, ventilated and some can even be used for chest drain insertion and other invasive procedures. The scope and complexity of the scenarios are much broader than with task simulators as the trainer can alter the parameters at will, choosing how the patient responds to any intervention. The simulation frequently involves a group of practitioners working together as a team, possibly from different disciplines and backgrounds, but in a realistic situation. Beyond simply teaching task mastery, these simulations allow trainers to assess a multitude of human factors including teamworking, leadership, decision-making, prioritisation, time-management and delegation skills. The simulation centre often has audiovisual recording equipment incorporated within it to allow detailed analysis of the simulation after it has finished, usually as part of the debriefing session, where the team review their performance with a trainer.

Advantages of simulation-based training

Patient safety – the concept that the first time a trainee can carry out a procedure is on an actual patient has become increasingly unacceptable to patients and trainers alike. Patients frequently ask junior doctor 'how many times have you done this before?' and trainers are rightly reluctant to put patients in harm's way if an alternative exists.

Organisational pressures – simulators allow trainees and trainers to engage in educational activity at times that are convenient to them, without needing to arrange for patients to be present. With task-based simulators trainees may wish to do a virtual procedure prior to an operating list to 'mentally rehearse'.

Standardisation – simulations can be standardised and repeated as part of OSCE examinations. Resuscitation is a frequently tested scenario, but as discussed earlier there are few limitations on what can be assessed, and scenarios designed to test specialised post-graduate skills can form part of continuing professional education.

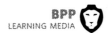

Repeatability – part of acquiring new skills is repetition and learning from mistakes. The ability to utilise these processes in a safe environment without recrimination or danger to patients is a powerful advantage of simulation. Trainers can devise scenarios with no solution and invoke and discuss the emotional aspects of losing a patient in spite of doing everything possible. This concept of debriefing is important and is something that trainees will need to continue throughout their years of practise.

Introducing new equipment or procedures and as part of continuing medical education – even experienced practitioners will need to be introduced to new equipment and procedures as medical practice continues to evolve. In the same way as the junior trainee can learn a new skill, simulation provides an opportunity for established practitioners to acquire new skills and enhance existing ones.

Research and development – with stringent ethical protocols in place to regulate research conducted on animals or human participants, simulation can provide a mechanism to test the feasibility of new techniques.

 Pause for thought
- How can you utilise high-tech simulation to advance training?
- Can you highlight specific areas within the curriculum where this could be incorporated?
- How could you assess the success and cost-effectiveness of simulation in your programme?

E-learning

As modern life evolves in step with technological innovations such as the internet, email, social networking and blogging it is not surprising that e-learning has become a significant component of medical education at both an undergraduate and post-graduate level. Different learners will utilise e-learning resources to differing degrees. For anyone engaged in e-learning and e-teaching, an

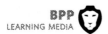

awareness of the technical abilities and computer literacy of your students is crucial in designing learning activities. Educators and students should be aware that much information on the internet is published in the absence of scientific scrutiny or peer review. While educators cannot be prescriptive about where their students should obtain information, the problem should be made clear and students should expect to defend any information they use to the same level as expected for paper-published information. Teaching students how to recognise reliable sources of information is especially important in the context of e-learning, and it is useful to have some suggestions where they might start.

Many universities and major medical journals have good peer-reviewed educational content available for public use.

Pause for thought
- How do you evaluate the quality of medical information?
- Do you apply different criteria to different forms of information and if so why?

E-teaching

E-teaching activities can be divided into absorb type, do type and connect type activities. These correlate to increasing advanced modes of learning outlined by Miller: knows – knows how – shows how – does. The table below gives example of each.

Activity type	Style of tasks	Examples of activities
Absorb type	Requires learner to read/ listen to or watch different media, may have an integrated assessment of factual knowledge (in the 'knows' realm of Miller's pyramid)	Online literature, case studies, narratives. Online recorded lectures and powerpoint presentations

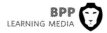

Activity type	Style of tasks	Examples of activities
Do type	Involves being able to demonstrate performance of a designated task. Uses online activity for the learner to participate in ('knows how' in Miller's pyramid)	Virtual laboratories and online experiments. Online clinical tasks such as prescription writing, fluid balance charts, death certificates. Virtual patients with simulated clinical signs or pathology
Connect type	Involves original work and thinking. Requires the learner to demonstrate new application for taught concepts ('shows how' on Miller's pyramid)	Problem-based learning and assessments Online reports or analysis including portfolios and logbooks of education aligned to specific goals

Table 10.1 E-teaching activities types

Any educational tool should be utilised optimally. With the multimedia resources available to e-teaching, the opportunity exists to present the same information in multiple formats (text or video for example) allowing trainees with different learning styles to access and use the same information in different ways.

When designing an e-learning activity certain criteria need to be considered.

Keep designs and accessibility simple and intuitive. The task should not test computer literacy and should be accessible to those with limited computer skills.

Utilise the strengths of technology by incorporating visual and audio recourse where they are beneficial over and above plain text alone. Incorporating multiple forms of information consolidates learning, but avoid unnecessary media that does not enhance learning.

Keep topics short and focused. As with traditional teaching, group content into related areas. This helps the learner appreciate how they are interlinked. Hyperlinking to related topics or references is a useful tool available to the e-teacher.

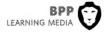

Align educational information to learning objectives and a specific curriculum. Building activities around an accessible online curriculum allows students to track their learning, especially if there is scope to record activities electronically ie logbooks, e-certificates for completion of modules etc.

This can be very useful as a way to collate evidence of learning for their regular educational review or to support revalidation when consultants.

Online activity is most powerful and effective when it accurately replicates real practice. As discussed earlier this promotes cognitive mapping, where the learning tool replicates real tasks with a high degree of felidity, thereby acting as a form of mental and practical rehearsal. Therefore tasks such as online prescribing, creating discharge summaries, performing patient coding on discharge and analysis of invasive monitoring (such as blood-pressure, CVP and ventilator tracings) lend themselves to online learning.

 Key points

- As advances in technology occur the ability for medical professionals to acquire new skills in a safe and more independent manner increases.
- By increasing the fidelity of the learning tools, transference of these skills to the clinical setting is enhanced.
- These tools are especially useful in rehearsing rare or high-risk events, but can equally be applied to most clinical tasks.
- Electronic media and online learning allow rapid dissemination of new medical knowledge, however caution about authenticity must be exercised.

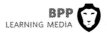

References

Kneebone R (2003) 'Simulation in Surgical Training: Educational Issues and Practical Implications', *Medical Education* 37: 267–277

Ziv A, Wople P, Small S, Glick S (2003) 'Simulation Based Medical Education – an Ethical Imperative', *Academic Medicine*, 78: 783–788

Savin-Baden M, Wilkie K (2007), A Practical Guide to Problem-based Learning Online (Abingdon: Routledge)

Useful links

Simulation and technology enhanced-learning initiative (STeLI), London Deanery (http://simulation.londondeanery.ac.uk/)

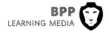

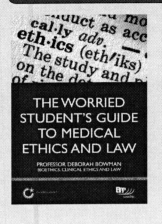

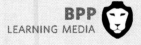

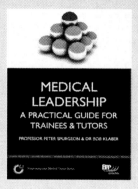
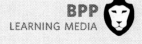

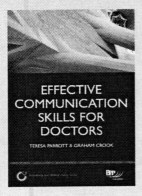
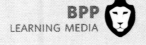

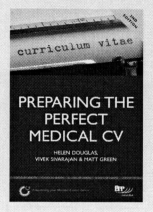
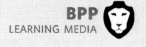

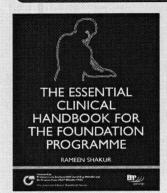
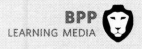

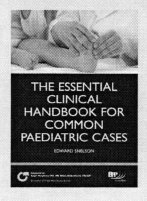
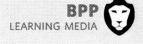

146

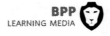